Natural Treatments
for
Fibromyalgia

AN *A* *to* *Z* Guide

By Kenna Simmons

Natural Treatments *for* Fibromyalgia

AN *A to Z* Guide

By Kenna Simmons

An Official Publication of the Arthritis Foundation

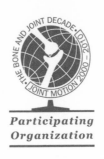

Participating
Organization

An Official Publication of the Arthritis Foundation

Copyright 2003
Arthritis Foundation
1330 West Peachtree Street
Atlanta, GA 30309

Library of Congress Card Catalog Number: 2003106549

ISBN: 0-912423-42-0

Printed in Canada

This book was conceived, designed and produced by the Arthritis Foundation. The mission of the Arthritis Foundation is to improve lives through leadership in the prevention, control and cure of arthritis and related diseases.

Editorial Director: SUSAN BERNSTEIN

Art Director: TRACIE BULLIS

Contents

Chapter III

All About CAM **52**

Contents *continued*

The A to Z Guide to

Natural Treatments for Fibromyalgia
and Other Chronic Pain Syndromes **72**

Acknowledgments

Natural Treatments for Fibromyalgia: An A to Z Guide is written for people with fibromyalgia and related diseases, as well as for their friends, family and loved ones. Bringing this book to completion was a team effort, including the significant contributions of dedicated physicians, healthcare professionals, Arthritis Foundation volunteers, writers, editors, designers and Arthritis Foundation staff. The editorial director of the book is Susan Bernstein. The art director and cover designer is Tracie Bullis.

Special acknowledgments should go to Kenna Simmons, the author of the book, who drew from her experience in writing about fibromyalgia from her days as Editor of the *Fibromyalgia Health Letter*. The chief medical editor of the book was John H. Klippel, MD, Medical Director of the Arthritis Foundation and former Director of the National Institute for Arthritis and Musculoskeletal Diseases at the National Institutes of Health. The book was reviewed for accuracy by Daniel J. Clauw, MD, Professor of Medicine, Division of Rheumatology, and Director, Chronic Pain and Fatigue Research Center; Interim Director, Center for the Advancement of Clinical Research; University of Michigan, Ann Arbor, MI; Don L. Goldenberg, MD, Chief of Rheumatology Service at Newton-Wellesley Hospital in Newton, MA; James McKoy, MD, Chief of Rheumatology and Pain Management at Moanalua Medical Center in Honolulu, HI; and Sherrie Piburn, who has had fibromyalgia since 1985, and has a degree in physical education.

*I*ntroduction

Fibromyalgia is a common – and often misunderstood – syndrome affecting as many as 3.7 million Americans today. There may be millions more people who have fibromyalgia and don't realize it, or have not yet been diagnosed. The first challenge for people with fibromyalgia is getting a diagnosis, but their challenges do not stop once they know the name of their condition. The real challenge for people with fibromyalgia is finding treatments that work to control pain, fatigue, poor sleep, muscle aches and other symptoms. The first treatments they probably try are medical, including prescription drugs like tricyclic antidepressants, analgesics, muscle relaxants or tranquilizers, or over-the-counter medications like topical analgesic creams or acetaminophen.

Unfortunately, many people with fibromyalgia say they do not find adequate relief from symptoms from the contents of a prescription bottle. They search for relief beyond what standard medicine has to offer, and enter the realm of natural treatments, also known as complementary and alternative medicine. Complementary and alternative medicine, often abbreviated as CAM, includes many different types of treatments, anything from the ancient to the innovative to the offbeat. The most important therapy for fibromyalgia treatment is regular exercise, and this practice should complement any course of therapy your doctor prescribes. In addition, relaxation techniques can offer great relief to people with fibromyalgia, lowering their stress levels and improving sleep.

Some CAM therapies included in CAM are age-old, herbal preparations that have much in common with contemporary drugs. Other therapies involve manipulating the body's tissues in specific ways to relieve pain. Still other practices within CAM are specific techniques for moving the body to improve its efficiency and flexibility.

If you are reading this book, you probably have a strong interest in CAM. Perhaps you are already using one or more CAM treatments and would like to know more about this area. Or, you may be eager to find new options for relieving pain and other symptoms of fibromyalgia that can complement the drugs your doctor prescribes. Or, you may be dissatisfied with the medicines you have been taking and wish to find other options. Whatever your situation, this book has valuable information for you about the many natural treatments for fibromyalgia. Use the book as a resource, but don't stop there. Talk to your doctor openly about your symptoms and your desire to know more about CAM therapies. Your doctor likely will help you find a way to integrate medical treatments with CAM, so you can find the right combination of treatments – the holistic approach, if you will – that works for you. Lifestyle changes, including exercise, diet and good health habits, can boost your well-being and help keep fibromyalgia symptoms in control. You are the most important player when it comes to managing your fibromyalgia. Your commitment to finding the right treatments, adopting a healthy lifestyle and maintaining a positive attitude is vital.

The Arthritis Foundation is committed to helping the millions of Americans with fibromyalgia. The Arthritis

Foundation offers several books and videos for people with fibromyalgia. The Arthritis Foundation's magazine, *Arthritis Today*, covers the latest news in fibromyalgia, including new research, drug treatments and health information. Our Web site, www.arthritis.org, contains up-to-date information on fibromyalgia research and treatments, as well as a message board where you can ask questions and discuss issues with other people with fibromyalgia.

Arthritis Foundation chapters nationwide offer helpful programs for people with fibromyalgia, including the Fibromyalgia Self-Help Course and exercise classes approved for people with the disease. In addition, the Arthritis Foundation raises money each year and allocates these funds to medical researchers searching for the cause of fibromyalgia and treatments that work to alleviate its symptoms. One day – hopefully soon – this research will yield the clues to the cure for fibromyalgia.

This book, *Natural Treatments for Fibromyalgia*, is an excellent resource for exploring natural treatment options for your fibromyalgia. It's a great place to start as you search for the therapies that will work for you. To learn more about fibromyalgia, consult *The Arthritis Foundation's Guide to Good Living With Fibromyalgia*, a book that goes more in-depth into the possible causes and many symptoms associated with this condition.

The Arthritis Foundation has several exercise resources either specifically designed for people with fibromyalgia or appropriate for people with fibromyalgia. *The Good Living*

With Fibromyalgia Workbook is a book full of useful guidelines for managing fibromyalgia, including exercise. Also available are the video *Let's Get F.I.T. (Fibromyalgia Interval Training)*, the two-video series *People with Arthritis Can Exercise (PACE)*, and exercise classes in most areas of the United States. Contact your local chapter for more information on fibromyalgia-appropriate exercise classes in your area. All Arthritis Foundation books and videos are available for purchase by calling (800) 207-8633, or on the Arthritis Foundation Web site, www.arthritis.org.

Chapter *I*
Understanding Fibromyalgia

To find helpful treatments for fibromyalgia, it is a good idea to begin by understanding what fibromyalgia is and what may be causing it to occur. This is no simple task, even for doctors. The exact cause of fibromyalgia is not completely understood by medical science at this time, and currently, the Food and Drug Administration (FDA) does not approve any drugs specifically for the treatment of fibromyalgia. But research has yielded some strong theories as the cause of fibromyalgia, what may happen in the body to cause pain and other symptoms, and how it may be treated with drugs, natural treatments and lifestyle changes.

What Is Fibromyalgia?

Fibromyalgia is a condition characterized by generalized pain and fatigue. It is included in the collection of diseases known as rheumatic diseases, but in contrast to arthritis, fibromyalgia pain can occur anywhere in the body, including the muscles, tendons and ligaments, rather than just the joints. Unlike arthritis, fibromyalgia does not damage joints or cause inflammation (which occurs when the body's immune system responds to injury, infection or disease, and can involve the destruction of tissue in the body). It is not a life-threatening illness, but it can be a debilitating condition to live with. When they are exhausted and hurt all over, people with fibromyalgia may have trouble completing even normal tasks of daily living. They may become depressed or angry, and may experience attacks of pain and fatigue that can leave them unable to function. There are many other symptoms that people with fibromyalgia experience (see p. 12), although the syndrome varies from person to person. No two people with fibromyalgia experience the same symptoms in the exact same way.

Fibromyalgia affects as many as 3.7 million Americans, although some experts feel the numbers may be higher. More women than men have the illness. It is the second most common rheumatic illness, after osteoarthritis, and it is often misunderstood. There is no lab test or X-ray that can diagnose fibromyalgia, and people with fibromyalgia often appear healthy. In fact, an added complication of fibromyalgia can be that friends, family, or co-workers (and even some doctors) don't believe you are sick. They may think you are being "too sensitive" or just pretending to be sick. That, of course, just causes additional anxiety and frustration for someone with fibromyalgia.

Because there is no marker that shows up on lab tests for fibromyalgia, it is diagnosed by its symptoms and by excluding other conditions. In 1990, the American College of Rheumatology, the official body of doctors who specialize in treating the musculoskeletal system, established its criteria for diagnosing fibromyalgia. Having fibromyalgia means you have the following symptoms:

- A history of widespread pain on both sides of the body, above and below the waist, present for at least three months;

- Pain in at least 11 of 18 tender point sites, and in all quadrants of the body if the length and width of the body were each divided in half.

Fibromyalgia Tender Points

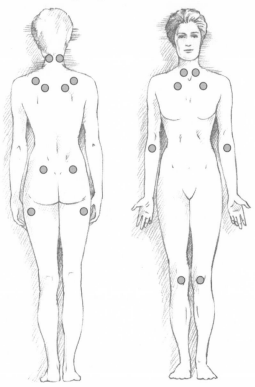

The dots in this figure indicate the various locations of tender points. People who have fibromyalgia experience undue tenderness when pressure is applied to many of these locations.

Tender points are areas of the body that are sensitive to pressure; the doctor will press on a tender point until his fingernail turns white (about nine pounds of pressure) and ask whether it hurts or not. Reactions may vary – some people with fibromyalgia cannot tolerate even the slightest touch, while others may feel pain only as the pressure increases. Although fibromyalgia is diagnosed by finding tenderness or pain at these specific points, people with fibromyalgia may experience pain or tenderness almost anywhere in their bodies.

THE HISTORY OF FIBROMYALGIA

For many years, fibromyalgia patients were told their condition was "all in their head." But fibromyalgia is not a new illness. Although the name for this condition was established recently, similar symptoms were described as long ago as the mid-1880s. In the early 1900s, the term "fibrositis" was used, and doctors assumed the tender points were caused by tissue inflammation. The word fibrositis means inflammation, -itis, of fibrous tissue, or fibro.

In 1989, Robert M. Bennett, MD, professor of medicine and director of the division of arthritis and rheumatic diseases at Oregon Health Sciences University in Portland, noted that the name was misleading, because fibromyalgia does not cause inflammation nor does it damage tissue. The following year the American College of Rheumatology decided to call the syndrome fibromyalgia, meaning "muscle pain" – a more accurate description of the condition. Fibromyalgia shares some symptoms (trouble sleeping, fatigue) with another condition, chronic fatigue syndrome. Researchers are not sure whether these two conditions are part of the same disease, are related, or are completely different conditions. Some people are diagnosed with both fibromyalgia and chronic fatigue syndrome. However, only fibromyalgia is diagnosed by a tender-point exam (see p. 22).

In addition to pain in the tender points and a history of widespread pain, most people with fibromyalgia report having moderate to severe fatigue, sleep disturbance, depression or anxiety, and other symptoms, although some of these symptoms are not included in the official diagnostic criteria. Many people with fibromyalgia report having other conditions that may or may not be related to fibromyalgia. While medical research has not proven a link between these many symptoms and conditions, some people with fibromyalgia also have:

- Irritable bowel syndrome (IBS), a condition marked by pain and alternating bouts of diarrhea and constipation;

- Restless legs syndrome, a condition marked by involuntary leg spasms during sleep or rest;

- Cognitive difficulties or "fibro fog," where the person may have trouble concentrating;

- Temporomandibular disorder, a condition marked by pain or stiffness in the face or jaw;

- Bladder irritability or bladder problems; and

- Muscular or migraine headaches.

People with fibromyalgia often undergo a number of laboratory tests to make sure their illness is not caused by other conditions with similar symptoms, such as thyroid conditions, that would require specific medication treatment. Despite the fact that fibromyalgia is not uncommon, it is unfamiliar to many people and even some doctors. Many people with fibromyalgia can spend years searching for a diagnosis. Once they receive a diagnosis, their journey has just begun: They will have to constantly explain their condition to people, and work with various doctors and health professionals to find treatments that work.

There is no known cure for fibromyalgia, but that does not mean that effective treatments don't exist. Many people find that fibromyalgia improves with treatment; for some, their symptoms may gradually disappear. For many people, fibromyalgia may be chronic, and these people need to find treatments that help relieve symptoms as well as coping methods that help them live with their condition.

Fibromyalgia symptoms can be treated with a variety of methods, including drugs, relaxation techniques, complementary and alternative therapies or CAM, and lifestyle changes such as better diet, regular exercise, stress reduction and pacing yourself in daily activities. Many people with fibromyalgia use a combination of conventional or allopathic medicine (such as prescribed drugs to help them sleep) and CAM. This combination is often described as integrative medicine. Some doctors have begun to embrace the concept of integrative medicine, and not only accept their patients' use of various CAM therapies, but guide them in finding the right CAM treatment, practitioners, supplements, and even performing or prescribing CAM therapies in addition to allopathic treatments. Not all physicians embrace this concept, however, and they may feel that CAM is either a waste of the patient's time and money or something that is secondary to medical treatment options. It's up to you to decide how to address the use of CAM with your doctor. We advise you to tell your doctor about any treatment you use, as many CAM treatments could have interactions with drugs your doctor prescribes. (We will discuss these in the A to Z section starting on p. 72.)

Chronic conditions such as fibromyalgia, for which conventional medicine has no cure at this time, can lend themselves to the integrative medicine approach. Integrative medicine combines mainstream medical therapies with alternative therapies that are safe and have been proven effective through scientific study. It is not an approach that suggests that you turn your back on medical treatment and embrace only alternative therapies, particularly those that are not carefully studied by scientists.

As more people turn to alternative therapies, research into these treatments by academic and scientific institutions such as the Harvard Medical School and the National Institutes of Health is increasing. The National Institutes of Health created a special institute to research these therapies, the National Center for Complementary and Alternative Medicine (NCCAM).

WHAT CAUSES FIBROMYALGIA?

The short answer is that no one knows what causes fibromyalgia. There are several theories about the cause of fibromyalgia and a number of scientific studies seem to show that different people develop fibromyalgia for different reasons.

Some studies indicate that exposures to different kinds of stress or injury, whether physical or emotional, can trigger the development of fibromyalgia. Neck injuries in particular seem to be associated with fibromyalgia. In 1997, researchers in Israel compared patients with neck injuries to those with leg injuries and found that fibromyalgia was 13 times more likely to develop after neck injuries. Other studies show that an infection or viral illness may sometimes precede the onset of fibromyalgia symptoms. [J Rheumatol 28:601-3, 2001]

Some scientists suspect that lack of exercise may contribute to fibromyalgia. For example, some individuals may need a certain level of exercise to produce enough of the body's hormones to keep from having pain and fatigue. Others suspect that the opposite, muscle overuse, may be a factor. For years, it was believed that fibromyalgia might be caused by a defect in the way muscles use energy. But in 1994 a study challenged that belief, finding that the muscles of people who are equally fit use energy in the same way, whether or not they have fibromyalgia.

Sleep disturbance is one of the symptoms of fibromyalgia, but some researchers believe it may also be a cause of the disease. Lack of restful sleep lowers the body's production of a growth hormone that is necessary for the repair of muscles. Sleep occurs in four stages; the first two are known as "alpha sleep" for the brain waves that occur during these stages, and the last two are known as "delta sleep." Delta sleep is essential to the body's ability to rejuvenate itself, because that's when a hormone, somatomedin C, is secreted. Somatomedin C helps the body repair muscle damage. People with fibromyalgia often don't get enough delta sleep, and may have lower levels of this crucial hormone. The interaction between sleep and fibromyalgia is discussed in greater detail later in this chapter.

There is a scientifically established link between depression and fibromyalgia, but no one knows whether depression is one of the things that cause fibromyalgia or if it is a result of the illness. Instead, it seems that all these conditions may contribute to fibromyalgia. Just as people with fibromyalgia experience symptoms in different ways, it appears that different people may get fibromyalgia for different reasons.

Researchers have also explored similarities between fibromyalgia and chronic fatigue syndrome, which is also characterized by muscle pain, sleep disturbance and persistent fatigue. Dr. Bennett has examined the relationship between fibromyalgia, chronic fatigue syndrome and myofascial pain, a fibromyalgia-type pain that is caused by injury and limited to only one or two parts of the body. (Two common forms are temporomandibular joint disorder, characterized by pain and tightness in the jaw, and repetitive strain syndrome, which causes muscle pain associated with repetitive tasks such as typing.) Dr. Bennett and others have come to believe that fibromyalgia may be at the high end of a spectrum of chronic pain, ranging from short-lived and localized pain at the low end to persistent, widespread pain at the high end.

WHY DOES IT HURT?

Promising research is being conducted concerning chronic pain. Some researchers believe that the central nervous systems of people with fibromyalgia process pain differently than the central nervous systems of other people. In people with fibromyalgia, this theory suggests, the central nervous system may become hyper-sensitive and interpret even ordinary stimuli (such as slight pressure) as painful. However, researchers don't know whether this sensitivity (called central sensitization) is a cause or a result of the chronic pain of fibromyalgia.

Several theories exist that suggest that people with fibromyalgia process neural hormones (chemical messengers of the central nervous system that influence sleep, pain sensation, the immune system, the constriction or dilation of blood vessels, and even emotions) differently than other people. Scientists have focused on substance P, which sends pain messages to the brain after an injury; serotonin, which regulates the brain's ability to control pain and mood; HPA hormones, which respond to stress; and growth hormones, which stimulate the growth and repair of bone and muscle.

SUBSTANCE P

The job of substance P is to transmit a message of pain to the brain. (The "P" stands for pain.) Studies have shown that the level of substance P in the spinal cord is three times higher than normal in people with fibromyalgia, suggesting that they may have a lowered pain threshold. A study conducted by I. Jon Russell, MD, of the University of Texas Health Sciences Center in San Antonio showed that the levels of substance P in the spinal cords of people with fibromyalgia remain high for weeks to months.

SEROTONIN

Serotonin affects the perception of pain, helping to "turn down the volume." It also promotes deep, restful sleep. Studies have found that levels of serotonin may be low or that the neurotransmitter may not be processed effectively in people with fibromyalgia. Decreased levels of serotonin may also lead to a change in the amount of substance P that is released (thus sending pronounced pain messages to the brain) and lower levels of stress hormones.

HYPOTHALAMIC-PITUITARY-ADRENAL (HPA) HORMONES

These hormones help affect the body's reaction to stress, and there is some evidence that people with fibromyalgia secrete these hormones differently than other people when faced with stress. Responses to stress can affect how the brain perceives pain.

GROWTH HORMONES

Growth hormones, which affect muscle function and are essential to the body's task of rebuilding itself, are largely produced during deep sleep. (See more on sleep in the next section.) Dr. Bennett has found that people with fibromyalgia have lowered levels of certain growth hormones than other people. These lower levels may leave muscles more vulnerable to trauma. When Dr. Bennett gave people with fibromyalgia daily injections of the growth hormone IGF-1, many of their symptoms improved.

It is still not clear, however, how the connections between hormone and neurochemical transmitter differences in people with fibromyalgia can be translated into specific treatments, or whether these connections point to a cause of fibromyalgia. People with fibromyalgia depend instead on individualized treatment to lessen their symptoms. There is no one-size-fits-all treatment. That's an important point to keep in mind when investigating alternative treatments. What works for one person with fibromyalgia may not work for another, and any treatment that claims to work for everyone should be regarded with suspicion.

SLEEP – WHAT GOES WRONG

Abnormal sleep patterns are a hallmark of fibromyalgia. Studies show that between 60 percent and 90 percent of people with fibromyalgia have sleep problems. Some find it hard to fall asleep, and they may wake up frequently during the night. No matter how long they stay in bed, they wake up feeling tired. Getting restful, restorative sleep is an ongoing challenge for people with fibromyalgia.

As we learned earlier, normal sleep involves four stages. Stage 1 is the transition from wakefulness to sleep (drifting off). Stage 2 is the first level of true sleep, where sleepers spend most of their time. During these two stages the brain sends out alpha waves, and these two stages are known as alpha sleep. Deep sleep occurs during stages 3 and 4, when the brain sends out delta waves. Without this deep "delta" sleep, people don't feel refreshed when they wake up, no matter how long they've slept.

People with fibromyalgia get little deep, stage 4 sleep. They have a higher proportion of alpha sleep, and alpha waves intrude on their delta sleep, waking them again and again. In 1975 Harvey Moldofsky, MD, of the Center for Sleep and Chronobiology at Western Division Toronto Hospital, completed an intriguing study showing that stage 4 sleep is fragmented in people with fibromyalgia. He also created the same abnormality in healthy people by waking them whenever they entered delta sleep; within a few days, these people developed symptoms of fibromyalgia. That has led some scientists to propose that sleep problems may be one of the causes of fibromyalgia.

Stage 4 sleep is crucial to the body's ability to restore itself. It allows the body to produce the growth hormone somatomedin C, which helps repair muscle. Dr. Bennett has found that people with fibromyalgia have significantly lower levels of somatomedin C in their blood than people without the condition, leading him to speculate that the muscles of people with fibromyalgia are not able to repair any of the tiny injuries that occur in muscles with everyday use.

Whether sleep disturbances are a cause or effect of fibromyalgia, many people find that their symptoms lessen dramatically when they improve the quality of their sleep. Drugs or alternative treatments and good sleep habits may help people with fibromyalgia get a better night's sleep.

DIAGNOSING FIBROMYALGIA

Getting a diagnosis of fibromyalgia can be difficult, because the symptoms of the condition are so diverse and because other illnesses have to be ruled out. In fact, a diagnosis of fibromyalgia is usually made after excluding any other conditions with similar symptoms. For someone with fibromyalgia, that can mean a series of seemingly endless screening tests. Be both patient and persistent! It can take a long time to get a proper diagnosis, given that you may have to wait for the results of many tests. But don't let your doctor dismiss your symptoms as normal aches and pains, or tell you that it's all in your head. If you encounter these kinds of responses, you may want to think about changing doctors or asking your primary care physician to refer you to a rheumatologist.

Your doctor may start with a thorough medical history, physical exam, and blood and urine tests. He or she also may order a series of X-rays. As people with fibromyalgia often experience numbness or tingling in their arms and legs, your doctor may order an MRI or CT scan to make sure a bone spur or herniated disc in your back is not causing these symptoms. In some cases, further blood tests are done to rule out autoimmune diseases (which occur when the body's immune system attacks its own tissue), such as lupus and rheumatoid arthritis.

Although many physicians do not believe it is necessary for a person to have 11 out of 18 tender points in order to have fibromyalgia, in many instances doctors will test for tenderness when they are considering this diagnosis. One way to do this is by performing a tender point count.

Tender points are areas of the body that are particularly sensitive to pressure. During a physical exam, your doctor will press lightly (just until the fingernail whitens) on 18 specific tender points as well as control spots and ask you if you feel pain. He or she will also ask you to rate the pain on a scale of one to ten. Tender points typically hurt only when pressed; sometimes people with fibromyalgia may not know they have tender points until a doctor applies pressure to them.

To provide a detailed medical history, prepare for your visit to the doctor by writing down important information. Some people find it helps to keep a diary of their symptoms. Your doctor may ask you these questions: Where are your symptoms? When did they start? Have they changed over time? How long have they lasted? Use the worksheet on the opposite page as a guide.

WORKSHEET
What To Tell Your Doctor

Thinking about your concerns before your appointment and writing them down to bring with you is a handy way to make sure that everything important to you gets covered. Think about these points before your appointment

When the pain started _____

What the pain feels like _____

_____

How long the pain usually lasts_____

Time of the day I feel the pain most _____

Other symptoms I've noticed _____

_____

Other medical conditions I have _____

_____

Childhood illnesses I've had _____

Adult illnesses I've had_____

Surgeries I've had_____

Medical conditions my family members have_____

_____

_____

You will also want to tell your medical doctor about any medications or treatments you use, including alternative therapies, dietary supplements and herbs, and over-the-counter medications. Even though your doctor did not prescribe alternative treatments, he or she should know everything you are taking.

Be candid with your doctor about any alternative medicines, such as herbs, supplements or alternative pain-relief techniques, you use. Your doctor needs to know the whole story in order to help you. Tell your doctor about any therapies you are considering, and share what you have read or heard about various therapies. Ask your doctor what he or she knows about any therapy you are considering. Although people think of alternative therapies as "natural," that doesn't mean they are automatically safe, and many herbs and supplements you can buy over the counter can have side effects such as drug interactions with other medications. Also ask your doctor to refer you to an established practitioner of alternative medicine or to write you a prescription; both actions will improve your chances of insurance coverage.

If your doctor objects to the treatments you propose, ask why he or she is opposed to them. Although many doctors are increasingly open to combining traditional and complementary medicine, not all of them favor this approach. In addition, some treatments may be a health risk for you. You should be able to have an open dialogue with your doctor about alternative therapies and their efficacy. Your doctor can help you avoid useless or dangerous treatments.

Handle your trip to the doctor as you would a business appointment. Come prepared, ask for what you need, and repeat what you hear. Have a list of questions you want to ask your doctor, and remember to be concise. Because you may be experiencing many symptoms, you may have a lengthy list that cannot be addressed in a single visit. Tell your doctor the reason for your visit and what you want him or her to do for you today.

CAM Considerations

- Be sure. Get an accurate diagnosis from your medical doctor first, so you know what you're treating.

- Be informed. The label "alternative treatments" can include everything from proven therapies to fads. Find out what scientific studies have been done on the safety and effectiveness of a particular treatment.

- Be scientific. In most cases it is unwise to add more than one new treatment at a time for fibromyalgia, because then it is difficult to tell if the treatment is working, and whether it has any side effects. Some doctors suggest that any new treatments for fibromyalgia should be approached in the same way: See if it seems to help and whether it has any side effects before deciding whether to keep using this therapy before moving to a new therapy. Sometimes it is even necessary to start and stop a therapy to tell whether it is working or not.

- If you are looking for an alternative medicine practitioner, ask your medical doctor for a recommendation or referral. If he or she is unable or unwilling to provide one, there are resources listed later in this book to help you find a practitioner.

- Never avoid or delay seeking medical treatment, or ignore advice from your medical doctor, because of something you have heard about complementary or alternative medicine therapies.

- Remember that improper use of these therapies can be dangerous.

- Think of alternative therapies as an addition to – not a replacement for – conventional medicine.

- Discuss any therapies with your medical doctor before making any decisions about treatment to avoid any dangerous interactions with other treatments.

Chapter **II**
Treating Fibromyalgia

With chronic conditions such as fibromyalgia, it is important for you to take an active role in your health care. Not only will it help you better manage your condition, it can give you a sense of control that can contribute to your overall well-being. Integrative medicine, which combines CAM and conventional therapies, is a multi-disciplinary approach that appeals to many people because it treats the patient rather than the disease – but for it to work, you must be responsible for the details of your own health care.

SELF-MANAGEMENT OF FIBROMYALGIA

What does self-management mean, exactly? It means that instead of being at the mercy of fibromyalgia, you actively manage your condition. Managing a chronic illness involves knowing your body and how it reacts to certain situations (stress, for example), medications and supplements, and even certain emotions (such as anger or frustration).

You can better manage your symptoms and lessen flares if you know your limitations and design a lifestyle to accommodate them: Making sure you have time to exercise and get a full night's sleep, learning to say no to things that tire or upset you, and communicating clearly with family, friends and even health-care providers about your condition. Self-management also means educating yourself about treatments for fibromyalgia – both conventional and alternative – and then, with your doctor's help, designing a management plan that works for you and sticking to it even when you don't feel like it.

While self-management does put more responsibility on you, the benefits are substantial. For one thing, when you take control of fibromyalgia, you start a cycle of emotional and physical improvement. Feelings of anger or fear will subside as you take control, and your overall quality of life will improve – which will lead to an improvement in your day-to-day functioning.

The goals of conventional and CAM therapies for fibromyalgia are the same: They seek to treat symptoms to improve quality of life. And there are several truly natural treatments which conventional medicine and alternative medicine agree should be the first line of therapy for someone with fibromyalgia. The first is exercise.

EXERCISE: THE BEST NATURAL THERAPY

When you are tired and hurting, the last thing you want to do is exercise. Besides, it seems counterintuitive: The more you move, the more your muscles hurt, right?

Actually, the reverse is true. Exercise is the best thing you can do for fibromyalgia. Reduced activity actually increases pain – going without exercise causes your muscles to become deconditioned, creating stiffness and increased muscle tension that leads to more pain. You have less stamina and get tired more easily. Aerobic exercise can also improve sleep quality, and raise the levels of serotonin and endorphins, both of which boost mood and lessen pain.

A 1999 study by Canadian researchers found that 41 fibromyalgia patients who participated in a six-week exercise and educational program showed significant improvement in their fatigue and pain. [Arthritis Care Res 1999 Oct;12 (5):336-40] Another study at the University of Missouri School of Medicine in Columbia showed that exercise lessened pain at tender points and improved physical conditioning. It was especially effective in conjunction with biofeedback and relaxation training. [Arthritis Care Res 1998 Jun; 11(3):196-209] Another study in 2002 examined the effects of a three-month program of aerobic exercises on 136 people with fibromyalgia. Participants were assigned to either an hour-long aerobic exercise class or a relaxation and flexibility class, which they attended twice a week. People in the exercise group had a greater reduction in tender point count, rated their symptoms much better and noticed that the effects lasted up to one year. [BMJ 2002 Jul 27; 325(7357):185]

If the idea of exercising seems overwhelming, remember there are many kinds of exercise, including low- or non-impact aerobic exercise such as walking, biking on a stationary bike or doing warm-water exercises that won't stress already painful muscles. The key is to start slow and gradually increase your workouts as your fitness improves. Gently stretching muscles before and after you exercise will increase your endurance and help avoid pain.

Your doctor may prescribe physical therapy, which can include an exercise program tailored specifically for you and monitored by a licensed physical therapist, along with pain-management techniques such as heat, ice, whirlpool, ultrasound, electrical nerve stimulation and biofeedback.

Two principles of treating fibromyalgia with exercise are to increase cardiovascular or aerobic fitness and to stretch, mobilize and strengthen tight, sore muscles. Though exercise may help reduce your symptoms, the exercise itself may not be pain-free, especially at first. You may experience cramping or fatigue in your muscles when you start, and even slow walking, for example, can cause more aches and pains. However, new pain that comes from new conditioning is not harmful; it may help to remind yourself that aches and soreness that may come from exercise are temporary and that you will feel better after a few days or weeks.

The key to exercise for people with fibromyalgia is to start slowly and to tailor any exercise to your age and fitness level. For example, you might start by walking five minutes two times a day, gradually building up to 45 minutes. If you get tired, take a break or slow down – but keep moving. Remember, any movement is better than none!

EXERCISE ESSENTIALS

A balanced exercise program includes three components: warm-up, strengthening and endurance (cardiovascular exercise), and cool-down.

> Warm-up Exercises: These can include some easy marching or arm swings before you exercise, or some range-of-motion (the range that your joints can move comfortably in a certain direction), stretching and strengthening

moves. Warm-up exercises safely prepare your heart and lungs for endurance, as well as help increase our flexibility and muscle strength. Some sample exercises are provided in this chapter. For some people, warm-up exercises may be the only ones they can do at first.

Endurance exercises: Swimming, walking, bicycling and even raking leaves are examples of endurance or low-impact aerobic exercises. Aerobic exercise is any activity that uses the large muscles of the body for a sustained period of time and increases the heart rate. These exercises help improve cardiovascular fitness and reduce fatigue. Build up gradually to these exercises – smaller, daily "doses" of exercise may work better than one large dose. However, it may be helpful to build up your endurance so you can work toward a goal of doing aerobic activity for a 30-minute session.

Cool-down exercises: As your exercise program gradually lasts longer, you need to build in a cool-down period to let your body lose some of the heat generated when exercising. A cool-down period helps relax your body, return your heart rate to normal and avoid sore muscles. To cool down, do your aerobic exercise in slow motion for three to five minutes, then do a few flexibility and strengthening exercises.

TYPES OF EXERCISE

To create a fitness program, you'll want to combine some flexibility and muscle-strengthening exercises with endurance exercises.

Flexibility/Stretching (Range-of-Motion) exercises: These exercises reduce stiffness and keep muscles and joints flexible. Your doctor or physical therapist can show you appropriate range-of-motion exercises and should be able to provide or direct you to illustrated exercises or appropriate exercise videotapes. Try to move your joints through their range of motion every day. Daily activities do not reliably do that and should not replace range-of-motion exercises.

Some range-of-motion exercises can help stretch or elongate the ligaments and muscles around your joints. The stretching helps maintain or improve the flexibility of those tissues, and it also reduces muscle tension. A sustained, non-painful stretch to a tight muscle can help relax that muscle, improving flexibility and reducing pain.

Strengthening exercises: These exercises help maintain or increase muscle strength. Strong muscles keep your body conditioned and better able to withstand the pain of fibromyalgia. These exercise will also help you better handle everyday activities such as climbing stairs or carrying groceries.

Two common types of strengthening exercises are isometric and isotonic exercises. Isometric exercises involve contracting a muscle with moving your joints – an example would be pushing one palm against the other. Isotonic exercise, on the other hand, does involve movement of your joints – an example would be straightening your knee while sitting in a chair.

Strengthening exercises must be carefully designed for people with fibromyalgia, but the payoff may be significant. A recent study suggested that strengthening exercises were more effective in lessening fibromyalgia symptoms than flexibility exercises. Knowing which muscles need to be strengthened and how to exercise without overstressing joints and muscles are key elements in a successful exercise program.

Endurance exercises: These exercises strengthen your heart and increase your lung efficiency. They also combat fatigue by giving you more stamina, so you can work longer without tiring. Endurance exercises also help you sleep better and control your weight. Almost any exercise that uses the large muscles in a continuous activity can be an endurance exercise. The signs that you are exercising at a level that will improve your conditioning are increased heart rate, increased breathing, and feeling warmer or sweating.

Some of the most beneficial endurance exercises for people with fibromyalgia are walking, water exercise and using a stationary bicycle.

WALKING

The great thing about walking is that it requires no special skill and it is inexpensive. You can walk almost anytime and anywhere, and you can easily monitor your progress. The only thing you need is a good pair of supportive walking shoes. A great guide to developing a walking fitness routine is the book *Walk With Ease: Your Guide to Walking for Better Health, Improved Fitness and Less Pain.*

WATER EXERCISE

Exercising in warm water is especially good for stiff, achy muscles. Warm water helps relax muscles and decrease pain, and the water also supports your body, putting less stress on hips, knees and spine. You can do warm-water exercises while standing in shoulder- to chest-high water or while sitting in shallow water. In deeper water, use a flotation device to keep you afloat. A water exercise program designed for people with fibromyalgia is *Let's Get F.I.T.*, produced by the Arthritis Foundation.

BICYCLING

Bicycling, especially on a stationary bike, improves fitness without putting too much stress on hips, knees and feet. When you begin, adjust the seat height so that your knee straightens when the pedal is at its lowest point. At first, don't pedal faster than 15 to 20 miles per hour or 60 revolutions per minute. Add resistance only after you have warmed up for five minutes, and don't add so much resistance that you have trouble pedaling. If cycling aggravates your pain, discuss this condition with your doctor.

WHEN YOU EXERCISE

Exercising regularly isn't easy even when you are in perfect health. When you have fibromyalgia, it's even harder. Here are some things to keep in mind when you exercise:

• Consult your doctor or physical therapist before you start a fitness program.

- If a form of exercise, such as walking, causes you increased pain that lasts two hours after you finish, slow down next time or make your workout shorter.

- If you find you can't do any form of exercise without significant pain, ask your doctor or physical therapist about a different form of exercise.

- Applying heat and cold may help lessen muscle aches. Heat increases blood flow, which can reduce stiffness, relax aching muscles and calm nerve endings. Apply no more than 20 minutes of heat (heating pads, warm showers, baths or whirlpools) to painful areas before exercise. Cold helps reduce muscle spasms and control pain. Apply no more than 10 to 15 minutes of cold (ice, cold packs or even bags of frozen vegetables) to painful areas after you exercise.

- Gently massage stiff or sore muscles before you exercise, and make sure you warm up.

- Don't do too much too quickly. Building endurance should be spread out over several weeks or months.

- Stop exercising if you feel dangerous symptoms such as chest tightness, severe shortness of breath, dizziness, faintness or nausea. If you experience these symptoms, call your doctor immediately.

- Use supports, such as elastic devices for elbows, knees and ankles. Use a walking stick or cane on your least affected side for stability and support. The handle should reach your wrist when your arm is by your side.

- Distract your mind while you exercise – listen to music, watch a video or exercise with a friend. Think about things you look forward to. Just keep your mind occupied with something besides pain.

• Think of your pain in a different way: a hot sensation, or a temporary discomfort. Remind yourself that as your muscles relax into the exercise, some of the pain will lessen.

DIET: EATING FOR HEALTH

Despite many rumors to the contrary, there is no "fibromyalgia diet." That is, no research has ever shown evidence that any particular food contributes to or lessens the symptoms of fibromyalgia. Some people with fibromyalgia notice their symptoms get worse when they eat certain things. Often the culprits are unhealthy foods everyone should avoid – fatty foods or foods loaded with sugar. If you suspect that a certain food makes your symptoms worse, eliminate it from your diet and then see if your symptoms improve.

Though there is no specific fibromyalgia diet, eating a healthy diet can help in managing fibromyalgia. It can also help you feel better, give you more energy, stay healthy, and prevent some diseases such as some types of cancer and cardiovascular disease. Eating a healthy diet also helps you avoid weight gain, which can worsen fibromyalgia symptoms. And it provides many of the vitamins and nutrients offered in some supplements, including anti-oxidants and fiber, which helps reduce symptoms of irritable bowel syndrome. Although supplements can help with certain symptoms of fibromyalgia, it's always better to get the vitamins and nutrients from fresh foods rather than processed pills. No supplement can make up for a junk-food diet.

Following a well-balanced diet means avoiding junk foods, fried foods and those high in sugar, and eating vegetables, fruits and whole grains. A healthy diet will ensure that your body gets the right amount of vitamins and minerals to combat fibromyalgia, and can help reduce the symptoms of irritable bowel syndrome.

THE CARBOHYDRATE QUESTION

You are probably familiar with the Food Guide Pyramid developed by the U.S. Department of Agriculture (USDA). This is a visual guide (shaped like a pyramid or triangle) to the daily diet suggested by the experts at USDA, including groups of foods and daily quantities of each you should consume. The pyramid is seen almost everywhere: It's emblazoned on food packaging, posted on the Internet and printed in magazines, books and brochures.

The Food Guide Pyramid was intended to provide healthy dietary guidelines by encouraging people to select most foods from the bottom of the pyramid and fewer from the top. Rice, bread, cereals and pastas were at the bottom of the pyramid, with 6 to 11 servings per day suggested. Vegetables (3 to 5 servings) were next, along with fruits (2 to 4 servings). Dairy products and meat (2 to 3 servings were next), topped off by fats and sweets, which were to be eaten only sparingly.

However, a 2002 study by the Harvard School of Public Health [Am Jour Clinical Nutrition, Dec. 2002] suggested an alternative diet that included less carbohydrates, favored whole grains over refined starches and made some distinction among protein and fats. The study found that participants who ate such a diet reduced their risk of chronic illnesses more than those who followed the food pyramid. The study didn't evaluate dairy products in the diet, nor did it establish daily recommended amounts for all food groups, so more research needs to be done.

What was intriguing about the study, however, was its emphasis on fats over carbohydrates. In the Harvard diet, "good" fats, such as olive oil, as well as the fats in nuts, seeds and many fish, would be consumed more often and refined starches less. Instead of getting protein from red meat, the Harvard diet suggests getting it from nuts and beans. A daily menu would look like this:

5 servings vegetables (potatoes do not count as a vegetable)

4 servings fruit

1 serving nuts or tofu

Eat white meat (fish or poultry) four times as often as red meat (beef, pork, lamb and processed meats)

3 to 6 servings whole grains, such as dark breads an high-fiber cereals.

The Harvard study doesn't suggest eliminating carbohydrates from your diet; indeed, our bodies depend on carbs for energy. But it does make a distinction between carbohydrates, separating these foods into two groups that have become known as "good carbs" and "bad carbs." "Good carbs" include fresh fruits, vegetables, beans and whole grains that are rich in fiber and whose nutrients are more slowly absorbed. That includes apples, melons, greens, carrots, cauliflower, beets, broccoli, green beans, spinach; whole-grain products such as whole-wheat or oat bread; brown and wild rice, oats; barley and millet. "Bad carbs" would include white bread, white pasta, white rice and potatoes, which are absorbed rapidly into the digestive system and cause blood sugar to spike. White rice, bread and pasta are made from processed white flours; much of the dietary fiber contained in wheat and rice is lost in this processing.

The bottom line on eating healthy? Consume more plant-based foods (fresh vegetables, fruits, beans, whole grains) and reasonable amounts of fish, poultry and low-fat dairy products, and limit your intake of red meat and foods high in sugar, salt or saturated fats.

BUILDING A HEALTHY DIET

Experts recommend five basic guidelines, which can be used to plan daily meals.

- Eat a variety of foods. That usually means eating more grains, fruits and vegetables than Americans usually do. A good diet includes choices from each of six food groups: breads and cereals, fruits, vegetables, dairy products, fats and meats. If you choose a vegetarian or vegan (no animal products like fish, meat, poultry, butter, eggs, milk or cheese) diet, make sure to get the protein you need from sources other than meat and dairy products. Vegetable protein can be found in foods like beans, nuts and soy foods such as tofu.

- Reduce fat and cholesterol. Cutting back on fat can help avoid heart disease. The American Heart Association recommends that people limit fat in take to no more than 30 percent of calories – about 67 grams a day or less for someone eating 2,000 calories. The AHA also recommends a cholesterol intake of less than 300 milligrams per day (about one and a half eggs). Look for "good fats" – polyunsaturated fats found in olive or canola oil, nuts and fish. Limit consumption of saturated fats, such as those found in butter or margarine, red meat, and coconut or palm oil.

- Eat more vegetables, fruits and whole grains. Carbohydrates have gotten a bad name lately, with many diets, such as the diet espoused by the late Robert Atkins, MD, advocating the near-elimination of carbohydrates from your menu. In reality, carbohydrates are necessary to supply energy to our bodies.

- Remember all carbohydrates are not created equal. Simple carbohydrates, such as the refined sugar found in a candy bar, supply few nutrients. While a candy bar supplies a quick boost of energy, it also raises blood sugar levels and puts stress on the pancreas, which produces insulin. Complex carbohydrates, on the other hand, come from fresh fruits, vegetables, beans, brown rice, and whole-grain breads and cereals. These carbohydrates are digested slowly and provide vitamins and minerals as well. (The high-protein, low-carbohydrate diets are right about one thing: Overeat any form of carbohydrate and your body will convert the excess to fat.)

- Spare the sugar and salt. Too much sugar promotes weight gain, not to mention tooth decay. When checking food labels for sugar, look for words such as dextrose, sucrose, fructose, honey and dextrin. As for salt, it causes your body to retain water and can affect your blood pressure. The American Heart Association advises holding sodium intake to about 2,700 mg a day, or about 1 1/4 teaspoon of salt. Check labels for sodium levels, especially in prepared and canned food.

- Drink alcohol in moderation. Alcohol is a depressant, but while alcohol may make you fall asleep, it can often lead to sleep that is disruptive and not restful. Some people may awaken after their body processes the alcohol and have difficulty falling back asleep. Alcohol also adds unwanted pounds and can promote tooth decay. Finally, alcohol can affect both traditional and alternative medications, so if you are taking any medications ask your doctor before drinking alcohol, even in moderation.

CAFFEINE

Caffeine, a common ingredient in many foods and beverages, not just coffee, is a powerful stimulant. Many people use caffeine to perk themselves up in the mornings, but too much caffeine can stimulate you too much and keep you awake at night. Because people with fibromyalgia often have trouble sleeping well, it's best to limit any caffeine to the early morning or, better yet, to avoid it entirely. Don't eat or drink anything with caffeine close to bedtime, and remember that some herbal teas and light-colored sodas contain caffeine. Check the labels carefully. Caffeine is also an ingredient in some weight-loss dietary supplements. Do not use these without discussing it with your doctor first.

A Final Word About Low-Carb Diets

While it's true that consuming too many carbs can make you overweight, a number of popular diets that encourage people to avoid carbs and sugar while eating fats and protein may just trade one problem for another. Yes, the typical American diet does contain too many simple carbohydrates and sugars, and eating healthy means cutting back on these items. But that doesn't mean eating instead large quantities of red meat and saturated fats, which are proven to increase the risk of heart disease, will be healthy. So while one of the low-carb diets may help you lose weight, if it doesn't advocate replacing simple carbs with more fruits and vegetables, it won't help your overall health. In the long run, you may tire of eating a restrictive diet of any kind, leading you to relapse and binge on the forbidden foods. Eating a balanced diet of moderate portions is the best approach.

The Diet Test

If you read about or hear of a special diet that claims to help fibromyalgia, ask yourself these questions:

- Does it favor only a few foods or suggest that you eliminate some food groups entirely? (The food groups are fruits; vegetables; carbohydrates such as breads and cereals; meats and/or nuts; dairy products; and fats.)

- Does it claim to cure fibromyalgia?
- Are its ads misleading, designed to look like news articles?
- Do its claims lack documented reports of scientific evidence?
- Do you suspect the diet could be harmful to your health?

If the answer is yes to any of the questions, avoid the diet. If you do suspect that certain foods make your fibromyalgia symptoms worse, talk to your doctor about your concerns or try removing the foods from your diet.

For More Information

Ask your doctor to refer you to experts in diet and nutrition for help designing a healthy diet, planning a weight-loss program or answering any questions. Local hospitals, health clinics and public health departments often have individual nutritional counseling available. Search for a registered dietitian or nutritionist in the phone directory, online or by asking your doctor for a referral. If your doctor prescribes this treatment, it may be covered by your insurance.

The Arthritis Foundation offers free information about diet and nutrition. You can call (800) 283-7800 to request information, including the brochure "Diet and Your Arthritis." The organization's Web site, www.arthritis.org, also posts information about diet, nutrition and arthritis-related conditions like fibromyalgia.

There are many reputable organizations that promote a healthy diet, offering information and guidelines for creating one. These organizations include:

American Heart Association – www.americanheart.org

American Cancer Society – www.cancer.org

American Diabetes Association – www.diabetes.org

American Dietetic Association – www.eatright.org

Some commercial weight-loss programs, such as *Weight Watchers*™ and *Jenny Craig*™, promote healthy eating and can offer benefits to someone looking to shed a few pounds. Each requires payment of fees, however. Before you sign on with any of these programs, check with your medical doctor first.

SLEEPING WELL

Many people with fibromyalgia find that medications help them sleep better. Among the sleep modifiers sometimes prescribed are zolpidem tartrate (*Ambien*) and temazepam (*Restoril*). There are also several supplements, such as valerian and chamomile, which may help with troubled sleep.

But there are also a number of things you can do to improve the quality of your sleep that don't involve taking any drug or supplement, beginning with eliminating any factors that contribute to sleep problems. Start by making your bedroom a restful, comfortable place, with a mattress and pillow that are right for you. Make sure it is not too hot or too cold, too noisy or too bright. Then

check to see if any of the following factors could be inter-
rupting your sleep.

DRUGS AND FOODS

Many drugs can interfere with sleep. Corticosteroid
drugs such as prednisone, which may be prescribed for
joint inflammation or allergies, can cause sleep difficulties, especially in high doses. Cold medicines that contain antihistamines, headache medications that contain
caffeine, and antidepressants such as *Prozac* can also
cause sleeplessness. Certain herbs and supplements can
also affect your sleep. Talk to your doctor about any
drugs, herbs or supplements you are taking and how they
may affect your sleep.

Caffeine in soft drinks, coffee and tea, including some
herbal teas and light-colored sodas, can cause insomnia.
Eliminate caffeine from your diet by switching to non-caf-
feinated drinks, and make sure to read all labels carefully to
see if a drink contains caffeine. There are now caffeine-free
versions of many popular soft drinks. Try one of these as a
substitute if you drink soda.

You've probably heard that you should drink eight
glasses of water a day. And it is important; water helps
flush out toxins in the body. But time your intake so that
you don't drink too much right before going to bed. If
you have to get up in the night to urinate, you may find
it hard to go back to sleep.

A heavy meal close to bedtime can keep you up, as can
indigestion resulting from a spicy or greasy meal. Watch

your eating habits to make sure you don't eat too much or eat the wrong kind of food. Take note of any foods or spices that may cause heartburn or indigestion. You may wish to avoid these foods or notify your doctor. If heartburn, chest pain or severe indigestion seems to occur often after you eat, notify your doctor. He or she may be able to treat this problem with medication.

If you smoke, stop. Not only does smoking cause heart disease and cancer, nicotine (the powerfully addictive ingredient in cigarettes) is a stimulant that makes falling asleep more difficult. If you smoke, ask your doctor for help in quitting. There are a number of programs and prescription treatments available to help you.

Drinking alcohol may help you doze off, but you may wake up after your body has processed the alcohol and have trouble getting back to sleep. Alcohol may seem to "relax" you, but it is actually a stimulant. It can keep you from having a restful night of sleep. Speak to your doctor about the amount of alcohol you regularly drink and ask if it may be interfering with healthy sleep.

Tips for Improving Sleep

- Maintain a regular daily schedule of activities, including going to bed and getting up at a regular time, even on weekends.

- Exercise, but not late in the evening.

- Set aside and hour before bedtime to relax. Try dimming the lights in your home abut an hour before going to bed.

- Create a dark environment for sleeping. Cover lighted clocks or nightlights if you find that the light bothers you or keeps you awake at times. Install shades, curtains or blinds designed to block all outside light if possible.

- Use your bedroom only for sleeping and being physically close to your partner.

- Avoid long naps. If you need a nap to get through the day, keep it short and schedule it well in advance of your bedtime.

- Take a warm bath before going to bed.

- Listen to soft music or a relaxation tape.

- Before you go to bed, write down anything you are worried about and make a to-do list. Then put it away for tomorrow so you can stop thinking about them.

- If you don't fall asleep within 30 minutes, or if you wake up in the night and can't get back to bed, get up and go to a different room. Try a relaxation technique, read or listen to soft music.

MANAGING STRESS

Stress can interfere with your ability to sleep, and it can cause or worsen flares. Having a chronic condition such as fibromyalgia can add a new set of challenges and daily adjustments that only increase your susceptibility to stress.

Stress is the body's physical, mental and chemical reaction to exciting, dangerous or irritating circumstances. Stress weakens the immune system, adds to anxiety and depression, and the body's physical reaction to stress (tensing muscles, for example) can exacerbate fibromyalgia symptoms. Unfortunately, no one can completely avoid stress. You can manage your reactions to stress, however, which will in turn help you manage fibromyalgia more effectively.

The key to managing stress is to make it work for you instead of against you. The following steps may help:

- Recognize your body's stress signals. Each person responds to stress differently. One person may get a headache, while another gets an upset stomach. By listening to your body, you can learn how stress affects you personally.

- Identify the cause of your stress. What causes you stress may not bother someone else, and vice versa. Once you know what the stressful aspects of your life are, you can decide how to change them, avoid them or adapt to them.

- Change what you can. Try to eliminate daily hassles when possible. Avoid places, people or situations that annoy you. Plan your schedule so that you aren't always caught in rush-hour traffic. Plan for special events: Instead of waiting to do gift shopping when everyone else is at the mall, shop year-round for gifts and put them aside until the holidays. If you're entertaining friends, buy prepared foods or make it a potluck dinner. Most importantly, don't be afraid to say no. Turning down extra, unnecessary duties even temporarily can reduce your stress. Don't sign up for a task that you don't think you can complete without stress. Let someone else volunteer if you don't feel up to it.

- Manage or accept what you can't change. Some situations can't be changed, but your point of view can. Think positively! Ask yourself if there is any hidden benefit to a stressful situation and make the most of it. Make sure you have a good support system, and use it. Talk to family, friends, clergy or others who are good listeners. And run a reality check on a regular basis – you may have to lower your expectations and standards. Is it really a crisis if the house doesn't get cleaned or the dishes aren't washed today?

- Adopt a lifestyle that resists stress. Set aside some time to relax every day. Relaxation is more than just quiet time; it is an active process to calm your body and mind that requires practice. You may want to try some mind-body therapies using guided imagery, yoga or biofeedback. All of these techniques are covered in the A to Z section, which begins on p 72.

Chapter III
All About CAM

Complementary and alternative medicine, or CAM, includes a wide variety of treatments and techniques. Not all treatments included in CAM are "natural"; some of these treatments involve chemicals, processing, machinery and other human intervention. So what makes a treatment part of CAM, or "natural," and what differentiates these treatments from traditional, allopathic or medical treatments? In many cases, the lines are blurred.

CAM usually includes supplements and herbal treatments not considered "drugs," items that are available without a doctor's prescription and not subject to the FDA for approval; exercise and movement techniques; therapies that fall outside the realm of allopathic medicine and may be considered "alternative" or "non-Western" in origin.

As noted before, some therapies usually considered alternative may be administered or suggested by your medical doctor, osteopath or other health-care professionals, such as physical therapists. Others may be administered or suggested by doctors of alternative medicine, including doctors of oriental or Chinese medicine, licensed acupuncturists, chiropractors and others. Insurance providers vary greatly on coverage of CAM therapies. You will have to consult your policy carefully to see if certain treatments are covered; most are not at this time. However, more insurance companies are covering services from chiropractors and other CAM practitioners, so this trend may be changing in favor of CAM proponents.

WHAT IS A NATURAL TREATMENT?

Whether you are investigating complementary and alternative medicine or you're already trying supplements to help with the symptoms of fibromyalgia, you're not alone. These therapies are exploding in popularity in the United States and around the world. In Europe, some CAM treatments are viewed the same as drugs and are prescribed by doctors.

Recent studies by Harvard Medical School indicate that some 42 percent of American adults – that's 82 million people – regularly use complementary therapies to treat common conditions. Alternative medicine can be especially appealing to people with chronic conditions such as fibromyalgia. While Western medicine is unsurpassed at treating acute illnesses such as infections and injuries, it has relatively few treatments for chronic conditions that may have more than one cause and take longer to treat. Western medicine is geared toward curing illness; when no cure is available, doctors and patients may have a hard time adjusting to that fact and "just" treating symptoms without a complete cure as a goal.

There's another interesting fact from the Harvard studies: Most of the people who responded said they used CAM in conjunction with (not as replacements for) conventional medical care. For years, many medical doctors were wary of or dismissive toward CAM therapies, because although these treatments may have had years of traditional use behind them, they weren't proven to work by scientific studies. But as CAM therapies are becoming more commonplace, more medical doctors are learning about CAM and some are integrating these therapies into their practice.

The mainstreaming of CAM has also led to scientific interest. The National Institutes of Health has established a National Center for Complementary and Alternative Medicine (NCCAM) that is funding clinical studies of CAM therapies to determine what works and what doesn't. The availability of valid scientific study findings may clarify the efficacy of some therapies and the uselessness of others; this data will also help doctors identify the most useful alternative treatments. A few therapies, notably chiropractic care, are sometimes covered by health insurance. Certain others, such as acupuncture or TENS, may be covered if your medical doctor writes a prescription for a specific therapy.

More patients are willing to discuss CAM therapies with their medical doctor, and that's advice you'll hear repeated throughout this book. If you choose to use a CAM therapy – whether it's acupuncture, herbs, dietary supplements or chiropractic care – talk to your medical doctor. He or she can watch for any drug-herb interactions that might cause side effects.

What's included in CAM? The NCCAM defines CAM as "medical practices that are not commonly used, accepted or available in conventional medicine." CAM therapies are not usually taught in medical schools and not used in hospitals. That's a pretty broad definition, and the terms used get even more complicated. CAM therapies may be called by a variety of terms, including alternative medicine, holistic medicine and unconventional medicine.

Many people think of CAM only as herbal supplements bought over the counter to treat various conditions. Even that can be confusing: Dietary supplements have actually been defined by an act of Congress (the Dietary Supplement Health and Education Act) as being a product taken by mouth that contains a dietary ingredient. That can include vitamins, herbs, minerals, amino acids, enzymes and metabolites. An herb, on the other hand, is a dietary supplement that is derived from a plant or part of a plant. In other words, herbs are dietary supplements, but not all dietary supplements are herbs.

Some supplements may be billed as natural treatments. It's important to realize that a "natural" treatment may not be natural at all – herbal preparations may be chemically processed, and some dietary supplements consist of enzymes made in a laboratory. And just because it's "natural" doesn't mean it's safe. Hemlock and arsenic are natural, but they are deadly poisons. While a prescription medication given to you by your doctor has been rigorously tested and certified by the FDA, supplements have not. They are considered food, not drugs. Even standardized preparations can have side effects, just like some prescription drugs.

If you choose to use a CAM therapy, then, you become responsible for your health care. That's not a bad thing. Many people, especially those with chronic illnesses, can gain a welcome sense of control by taking a more active role in their own care, whether CAM or conventional. This does mean that you have to work a little harder, do some research on the therapies you choose, ask a lot of questions and make informed decisions.

A Few Terms to Know

Allopathic or Western medicine – Medicine practiced by holders of M.D. (doctor of medicine) or D.O. (doctor of osteopathy) degrees and allied health professional (registered nurses, physical therapists, psychologists). Also called mainstream or conventional medicine

Alternative – Often used to refer to CAM therapies used by themselves in place of conventional medicine

Chinese medicine – A form of alternative therapy that treats disease or illness by focusing on the whole person, rather than a specific symptom. Herbs, acupuncture, massage, and qi gong may be used in treatment.

Chiropractic – A type of treatment that seeks to relieve back pain by manipulating the spine. Some chiropractors also believe that spinal adjustments can cure disease or alleviate other conditions such as high blood pressure, migraines and symptoms of fibromyalgia, but there is no evidence to indicate this is true. Chiropractors are not medical doctors and cannot prescribe drugs or perform surgery.

Complementary – Often used to refer to CAM therapies used in combination with conventional treatments

CAM – Complementary and alternative medicine, defined as medical practices that are not commonly used, accepted or available in conventional medicine. Also called alternative medicine, holistic medicine or unconventional medicine

Dietary supplements – A product intended to supplement the diet that contains one or more of the following ingredients: a vitamin, mineral, amino acid, enzyme, herb or other plant, or a concentrate, metabolite, constituent, extract or combination of any of these ingredients, intended for use as a capsule, powder, softgel or gelcap. Supplements are considered food, not drugs.

Herbal medicine – A preparation derived from a plant

Integrative medicine – The combination of conventional mainstream medical therapies with CAM therapies for which there is scientific evidence of safety and effectiveness. Also refers to medical doctors who incorporate CAM into their practice

Osteopathy – Osteopathy requires the same training as allopathic medicine (practitioners are medical doctors), but places more emphasis on treating the whole person and associates illness with disorders of the musculoskeletal system.

THE FACTS ABOUT CAM

Because there is no cure for fibromyalgia, the goal of CAM therapies and conventional medicine is the same: to treat your symptoms. Before you choose a CAM therapy, make sure you understand its risks and possible benefits. Because CAM therapies, particularly herbs and supplements, don't have to follow the same rules that prescription medications do, you'll need to do a little research. Common sense helps: If a supplement is promoted as a cure-all, or a cure for fibromyalgia, it's a fraud. Be skeptical – if it sounds too good to be true, it probably is.

The first step is evaluating a therapy's safety and effectiveness. Although scientific research on CAM is fairly new and may not be available for every therapy, it's the place to start. Don't trust something you see on a Web site or read about in an advertisement, or something you hear about from a friend. One way to get scientific information about CAM therapies is to ask your medical doctor. Tell them about the therapy and ask about its safety or interactions with any medications you may be taking. If your doctor does not know about the therapy, he or she may be able to refer you to someone else, or to help you interpret any scientific articles you have found about the therapy.

You can use the Internet to search for articles, but make sure they come from a trusted source. One excellent database that gives summaries of scientific studies on complementary and alternative treatments is called CAM on PubMed, found at www.nlm.nih.gov/nccam/camonpubmed.html. Developed by NCCAM and the National Library of Medicine, it is easy to use and all the articles are peer-reviewed – the gold standard of medical research, where other researchers in the same field have reviewed the article and found it to contain accurate data. Another database, International Bibliographic Information on Dietary Supplements (IBIDS), is not as easy to navigate and users can experience long waits, but the information is solid. It is found at http://ods.od.nih.gov/databases/ibids.html.

Two other databases provide substantial information about herbs and supplements, but each requires a hefty subscription fee. The Natural Medicines Comprehensive Database (www.naturaldatabase.com) contains information about more than 1,000 herbs and supplements and includes an extensive list of scientific studies about each one; it costs $92 for a year's access to the database. Natural Standard (www.naturalstandard.com) aggregates evidence-based information about alternative treatments, including herbs and supplements. All information then undergoes peer review. A year's subscription costs $99.

NCCAM recommends the following checklist for evaluating information on the Web:

- Who runs the site? A reputable Web site makes it easy for you to see who is responsible for the site's information, with clearly marked logos on every page.

- Who pays for the site? Does it accept advertising? Is it sponsored by a supplement manufacturer?

- What is the purpose of the site? Look for an "About us" or "About this site" link. The purpose should be clearly stated and help you evaluate the reliability of the information.

- Where does the information come from? Many sites include articles or abstracts from other sources; the original source should be clearly labeled.

- What is the basis of the information? Facts and figures should reference medical studies or research, such as articles in scientific journals, and opinion or advice should be clearly differentiated from facts.

- How is the information selected? Do people with scientific training review the material? Is there an editorial advisory board?

- How current is the information? Material should be dated, and any citations from medical journals should also carry publication dates.

- How does the site choose links to other sites? Some link to sites that meet certain standards, others accept paid links without review.

- How much information does the site ask you to provide? Some sites may ask you to subscribe or become a member. If that's the case, the site should clearly state its privacy policy and tell you what it plans to do with any information. Make sure a site is secure before offering any personal or credit card information over the Internet.

- How does the site manage interactions with visitors? Is there a way for you to contact the site's owner? If the site hosts chat rooms or forums, are they moderated?

After you've done some research, you can evaluate the evidence and determine if you want to choose a particular

CAM therapy. You may decide to choose a certain therapy even if the evidence is unclear, but you will have a good idea of the risks involved and how to determine of the treatment is working for you. Always tell your medical doctor that you are trying a CAM therapy, so he or she can watch for side effects and interactions. If, after you have talked with your doctor about CAM, he or she advises against the therapy, ask for a detailed explanation. If your doctor refuses to consider CAM, you may want to search for a doctor who practices integrative medicine. Above all, don't be dishonest with your doctor about using CAM therapies.

CAM Red Flags

Choose another therapy if:

• You cannot find published studies about the effectiveness of a particular therapy in reputable scientific journals;

• The vendor or practitioner claims the product or treatment works by a secret formula;

• The therapy is touted as a "cure" for fibromyalgia;

• The therapy is advertised only by direct mail, infomercials, Web sites or ads that pretend to be news stories; real therapies are reported in medical journals;

• The only proof comes from testimonials from satisfied customers; and

• The vendor or practitioner does not want you to see a medical doctor.

Is CAM Safe?

You may wonder if it is safe to use complementary and alternative therapies. The answer is, it depends. Some CAM therapies have been used for hundreds of years and have a well-developed tradition of effective use, while others are new and not much information exists. That's why it's so important for you to be an informed consumer, particularly when it comes to herbs and other supplements that you can buy without the advice of your doctor or a pharmacist.

To work, herbs and supplements must have an effect on the body, and they must be consumed in amounts that cause a physical reaction. In that sense, they are no different from drugs. Chances are, anything that fits that bill can also be dangerous if misused. Some supplements are dangerous by themselves: The herb comfrey has been linked to liver damage and cancer, the supplement ephedra (also sold as ma huang) to sudden death, and the herb kava to liver damage. Other supplements can interact with prescription drugs, over-the-counter medications and other herbs. St. John's wort can interfere with the effectiveness of birth control pills; ginkgo and ginger can interact with warfarin (*Coumadin*) or aspirin. Ginkgo and other herbs increase the risk of bleeding and should be stopped before any surgery.

That's why it's so important to talk to your medical doctor about any CAM therapy you are considering, and to gather as much reputable information as you can. Here is a list of information to look for:

- Find out what the benefits of the therapy will be.

- Identify the risks associated with the therapy.

- Consider whether the benefits outweigh the risks.

- Identify the side effects that may occur.

- Find out if the therapy will interfere with other treatment or interact with any medications you take.

Finally, see if the therapy will be covered by health insurance. Some, such as chiropractic and acupuncture, may be covered, but supplements likely are not and can be expensive.

Your pharmacist can provide on-site information or advice about herbs and supplements sold in pharmacies or supermarkets with pharmacists on site. If you are interested in trying an herb or supplement, consult the pharmacist before selecting a product.

WHAT YOU NEED TO KNOW
ABOUT SUPPLEMENTS

The safety of a CAM product, such as a supplement, sold over the counter depends on several things: its ingredients, where those ingredients come from, and how they were processed. The supplement's manufacturer is responsible for making sure the product is safe before it is sold. The FDA does not require testing of supplements, though it can ban the sale of products shown to be dangerous. In addition, if the product's label claims to treat, cure or prevent a disease, the product is considered to be an unapproved drug and is being sold illegally. That's why the labels on reputable dietary supplements have a disclaimer.

The advice when you're choosing a supplement is the same as when you're considering any CAM therapy: Do your research. Are there scientific evidence and clinical studies (not just testimonials) to back up the supplement's claim? It is important to note that at this time, there is very little scientific evidence to back up the effectiveness of most CAM therapies. Check out the manufacturer's Web site to see what research is listed. Look for articles published in scientific journals, not testimonials from individuals, even doctors.

See what the federal government says about the supplement. You may have to do a little surfing. The Web sites aren't always easy to use and some search functions work better than others, but it's worth it.

Here's a quick guide to some informative sites:

- The FDA's Web site includes a Center for Food Safety and Applied Nutrition section on dietary supplements at www.cfsan.fda.gov.

- Product recalls and safety alerts are found at www.fda.gov/opacom/7alerts.html (supplements are listed along with a variety of other products).

- The Federal Trade Commission also maintains a list of fraudulent claims and consumer alerts at its Diet, Health and Fitness Consumer Information site, www.ftc.gov/bcp/menu-health.htm.

Watch for misleading language from the manufacturer: "miracle cure," "exclusive formula," "what your doctor doesn't want you to know," or claims that the supplement cures a variety of unrelated conditions. These are warning signs of fraud.

Once you have investigated a supplement, you'll face another choice: which brand to buy. Supplements are available at drug stores, grocery stores, on the Web, at health clubs, at special stores and through mail order. Because the FDA doesn't test supplements, there is no guarantee that the supplement will actually have the amount of active ingredients claimed on the label or that the substance is pure. Independent testing has often found that brands vary in the amount of active ingredients they contain. One independent lab conducted a study of seven national brands of St. John's wort for the *Boston Globe* and discovered only one contained the amount of the active ingredient hypericin claimed on all the product labels. Contamination during the manufacturing process poses real risks: In the 1980s, contamination of the supplement tryptophan led the FDA to ban the substance after several people died.

How do you know which products to choose? First, look for the USP (United States Pharmacopeia) symbol on the label. The USP sets standards for manufacturers of drugs and supplements, and the symbol indicates that a supplement has met USP standards for strength, purity, packaging and labeling, that it has an FDA- or USP-accepted use, and that it will dissolve or disintegrate in the body. Another symbol to look for is the NF (National Formulary) mark, indicating that a supplement meets USP standards but does not have an FDA or USP accepted use. Neither symbol proves that a supplement is effective, just that it meets minimum manufacturing standards.

All manufacturers of supplements are supposed to follow standards for food processing, known as Good Manufacturing Standards, which ensure the quality will not vary from batch to batch. Some adhere to the higher standards set for prescription drugs, and will say so on the label.

To be sure you know what you're getting, choose single-supplement products that show how much of the active ingredient is in each dose. This also makes it easier for you to determine which ingredients are effective, and to calculate side effects and interactions.

How to Choose a CAM Practitioner

Finding a health-care practitioner, whether a medical doctor or a CAM practitioner, is crucial to ensuring that you receive the best treatment available. To find a CAM practitioner, the first place to start may be your medical doctor. Ask if he or she can recommend someone or make a referral. This can also help your chances of having a CAM therapy covered by health insurance.

You can also contact a hospital or medical school to see if they have a list of CAM practitioners. They may even have a CAM center. In addition, some medical doctors also include CAM therapies as part of their allopathic practice. These doctors practice integrative medicine (see p. 69) and may be able to suggest supplements or perform alternative treatments such as acupuncture. Some physical therapists (PTs) also perform some alternative treatments, such as massage therapy.

You can also contact a professional organization for the type of CAM therapy you seek (some organizations are listed after the therapies in this book). Your state may have a regulatory agency or licensing board for some kinds of practitioners and can provide you with a list of members. A number of states license acupuncturists, chiropractors, homeopaths and massage therapists.

Your health insurance organization may be a source of lists for CAM practitioners whose therapies are covered. Finally, you can ask someone you trust who is knowledgeable about CAM to suggest a practitioner.

Once you have the names of several CAM practitioners, you'll want to gather some information on each. Contact the practitioners on your list and ask for a consultation either in person or by phone. There may or may not be a charge; ask about fees while you are making the appointment. Ask them the following questions:

- What training or qualifications do you have? Do you have experience treating someone with fibromyalgia?

- Do you have a good understanding of fibromyalgia? Have you treated other patients with fibromyalgia?

- Do you believe this therapy can be effective for fibromyalgia? Is there any scientific research that supports that belief?

- How many patients do you usually see in a day? How much time do you spend with each?

- Do you have a brochure or Web site that can give me more information?

- How much do treatments cost? Do you accept my health insurance?

- What will happen during my first visit?

- Can you tell me now what the estimated length of treatment will be? Will I have to come back for a series of treatments? If so, how many? How will I be billed?

- How will this therapy complement my conventional medical treatment? Will you work with my medical doctor during my treatment?

When you have selected a CAM practitioner, prepare for your first visit. The practitioner will want to know about your health history and any prescription drugs, vitamins or supplements you take. You will want to ask questions, too, to find out more about the suggested therapy, its benefits and risks, and what possible side effects you can expect.

Find out if your treatment will interact with any conventional medical treatment, and whether there are conditions for which the therapy should not be used. After the visit, evaluate your reactions: Was the practitioner easy to talk to? Did the practitioner seem knowledgeable about fibromyalgia, and did the suggested treatment seem appropriate to you?

In the following sections, we'll learn more about the many natural treatments for fibromyalgia.

Integrative Medicine: A New Path

Whatever choices you make about using CAM therapies, you can benefit from getting advice from a doctor who neither automatically advocates nor summarily dismisses use of CAM therapies. Exploring CAM under the guidance of a medical doctor is the safest way to go about it.

Don't assume your doctor is negative about CAM. Ask your doctor to discuss the benefits and risks of CAM before you go to a practitioner. Talk honestly with your doctor about why you are seeking this therapy. Your doctor may be able to provide a referral.

Ask your doctor what he or she knows about a particular CAM therapy, and listen to the answer. Always tell your doctor about any CAM therapy you are trying, whether it is taking a supplement, performing special exercises, or seeing a CAM practitioner.

If you are satisfied with your medical treatment but your doctor refuses to talk about CAM, you may need to consider how important CAM is to you. You may decide to get a second opinion or even to change doctors. If you do, look for a medical doctor who is open to talking about CAM.

Remember:

- Do not rely only on a CAM practitioner for your medical care.

- Never halt your medical doctor's treatments, such as drugs or prescribed exercises, just because a CAM practitioner advises you to do so. This could be dangerous.

- Try contacting a hospital or medical school to find a doctor who practices integrative medicine in your area. The American Holistic Medical Association also lists MDs, DOs and licensed health-care professionals who take a holistic approach to health care. Contact the organization at (703) 556-9327 or on the Web at www.holisticmedicine.org

The A-Z Guide to

Natural Treatments for Fibromyalgia
and Other Chronic Pain Syndromes

In this section, we will explore the many complementary, alternative and natural treatments available for fibromyalgia, chronic pain and conditions related to fibromyalgia.

The treatments are organized alphabetically. Each entry includes the following:

- Official and common names of the treatment;

- Common uses of the treatment;

- Scientific name when applicable;

- Basic description of the treatment and its history;

- Scientific evidence concerning its efficacy;

- Possible side effects or interactions;

- Safety concerns; and

- Typical dosage.

References of the sources of scientific evidence are provided; these notations refer to the scientific or medical journals where the studies were reported and published.

Based on current evidence, a few of the treatments listed here may be dangerous or best avoided. These treatments will be marked with a special "warning" icon:🔞. It's important for you to talk to your doctor before trying any of the treatments listed here. Dosage and instructions may vary greatly from person to person, depending on your current health, weight, other medications you take and other factors. Your pharmacist can also discuss the benefits and risks of many herbs and supplements, and advise you about the various brands of supplements available in drugstores and pharmacies.

In the end, the decision about whether or not to use one or many of these treatments rests with you. It is up to you to be informed, to stay up to date on new research and warnings, to decide what investment of time or money you are willing to make, and what risks you are willing to take when it comes to using natural treatments. You will have to do your homework. This book offers you only one guide to help you begin your task of finding worthwhile treatments for your symptoms.

Natural treatments can include many different types of therapies. Some are herbs and supplements that, like medicines, are swallowed, eaten or rubbed on the skin. Others involve a practitioner manipulating your body's tissues and joints, using instruments on your body, or helping you learn to move in less painful ways.

Throughout the A to Z section of this book, we have placed special symbols next to each entry to help you differentiate between them, and also to see what treatments are considered potentially dangerous. Use this key to understand these symbols:

 These treatments are herbs or supplements, including those in natural, pill, liquid, cream or tincture form.

 These treatments involve manipulation of your body's tissues and joints, or new philosophies of movement and mind-body healing.

 Warning! These treatments are potentially dangerous and should be avoided.

5-HTP; 5-Hydroxytryptophan

Common uses:

Treating depression, weight loss, anxiety, fibromyalgia

5-HTP is derived from the amino acid tryptophan and used by the body to make serotonin, a neurotransmitter that affects mood and well-being. The body converts tryptophan, found in high-protein foods such as beef, chicken and fish, into 5-HTP and then into serotonin. 5-HTP supplements are made from the seeds of Griffonia simplicifolia, a plant found in Africa.

Because 5-HTP may boost serotonin levels in the body, it has been proposed to treat depression and anxiety, as well as a variety of conditions such as fibromyalgia that are linked to low serotonin levels.

Experts disagree about the safety of 5-HTP because of its relation to tryptophan. In 1989 the Food and Drug Administration banned tryptophan (often sold as L-tryptophan) when some people who used the supplement died and others developed a blood disorder called eosinophilia-myalgia syndrome (EMS) after taking it. The Centers for Disease Control and Prevention determined that contamination during the manufacturing phase was responsible. Although 5-HTP is produced differently, there are still concerns about contamination (see Safety Concerns on p. 78), making it potentially dangerous to take.

In addition, 5-HTP interacts with many drugs and supplements. Ask your doctor or pharmacist for more information.

SCIENTIFIC EVIDENCE

Many studies have suggested that 5-HTP may be an effective treatment for depression, with fewer side effects. The best study compared 5-HTP to fluvoxamine (*Luvox*), a selective serotonin reuptake inhibitor (SSRI) similar to fluoxetine (*Prozac*). Participants showed a slightly higher overall decrease in depression, and 5-HTP appeared to act more quickly than the SSRI. [Psychopathology 1991; 24(2):53]

5-HTP has also been studied for fibromyalgia. One double-blind study found that people with fibromyalgia who received 5-HTP saw improvement in all symptoms, including pain, stiffness, sleep quality, anxiety and fatigue, vs. placebo. [Jour Int Med Res 1990; 18 (3):201]

A few studies have also suggested that 5-HTP may improve sleep quality in healthy individuals as well as those with insomnia, but the research is not clear. Likewise, a few studies have suggested that 5-HTP may promote weight loss in overweight women, but more research is needed.

SIDE EFFECTS AND INTERACTIONS

- 5-HTP generally has few side effects, but some can be serious. For that reason, you should not take 5-HTP unless supervised by a medical doctor.

- Some people experience stomach upset, nausea, gas or bloating, diarrhea, anorexia, drowsiness and dry mouth.

- 5-HTP may lower cholesterol and blood pressure, cause the body to retain sodium and slow the heart rate. If used for long periods of time, 5-HTP may cause seizures.

- Cases of EMS have been associated with 5-HTP

- The combination of 5-HTP with antidepressants can magnify the effects of the drugs and boost serotonin levels too high, causing a condition known as serotonin syndrome. It is characterized by confusion, anxiety, sweating, rapid heart rate and muscle spasms. Do not take 5-HTP with any antidepressant, such as fluoxetine (*Prozac*), phenaline (*Nardil*), amitriptyline (*Elavil*), trazodone (*Desyrel*), or venlafaxine (*Effexor*). Also avoid taking 5-HTP if you take tramadol (*Ultram*) or sumatriptan (*Imitrex*).

- In theory, St. John's wort, SAMe, vitamin B6, niacin and magnesium can increase the side effects of 5-HTP. Use caution if you combine these supplements.

- Do not take 5-HTP if you have Parkinson's disease or scleroderma.

- Do not take 5-HTP if you take carbidopa, a drug prescribed for Parkinson's disease and restless legs syndrome.

- Pregnant and breast-feeding women should avoid 5-HTP.

SAFETY CONCERNS

- 5-HTP was thought to avoid the contamination that resulted in several deaths from tryptophan and led the FDA to ban the supplement. However, in 1998 Mayo Clinic researchers found peak X, the same contaminant found in tryptophan supplements, in some 5-HTP supplements.

- Manufacturers of 5-HTP are now supposed to screen for any sign of peak X, and the FDA has not issued any further warnings about 5-HTP. Pay attention to any reports that follow up on contamination of 5-HTP.

• If you choose to take 5-HTP, do so under the supervision of a medical doctor. Ask your doctor to monitor your eosinophil levels (white blood cells involved in immune response).

DOSAGE

A suggested dose of 5-HTP is 50 mg to 100 mg three times daily. Start with a small dose possible to minimize the danger of side effects.

Acupuncture

Common uses:
To treat nausea caused by anesthesia or chemotherapy; dental pain; addiction; headache; menstrual cramps; fibromyalgia; myofascial pain; osteoarthritis; lower back pain; carpal tunnel syndrome; asthma

Acupuncture, a type of traditional Chinese medicine, is one of the most ancient and widely used treatments in the world. In acupuncture, extremely thin, solid needles are inserted into the skin at certain points on the body to relieve pain and nausea.

Acupressure and moxibustion (the burning of herbs on or near the skin) are variations on the technique. Some practitioners also stimulate the needle points electronically (called electroacupuncture).

According to traditional Chinese medicine, all organs of the body are related. Acupuncture points connect with meridians, or pathways, that conduct *qi*, which is the energy or life force that flows throughout the body according to traditional Chinese medicine. Qi (pronounced "chee") is influenced by the opposing forms of yin and yang, which maintain balance in the body. When this balance is upset and qi is blocked, the body becomes ill. Acupuncture works by removing any blockages of qi and restoring the normal flow of energy.

Though studies have shown that acupuncture is effective for some people, scientists don't know why. They theorize that acupuncture points may stimulate the body's central nervous system, causing it to release pain-killing endorphins or other brain chemicals that reduce pain.

SCIENTIFIC EVIDENCE

Some studies show that acupuncture is helpful in relieving both chronic and sudden pain, though other studies show it is not as effective for chronic pain. However, a recent study in Brazil examined the use of acupuncture in the treatment of fibromyalgia and found that it significantly reduced both pain and depression. [Rheumawire 11/22/02] The study also found that benefits from acupuncture, which was administered once a week, started about two to three weeks into treatment and reached its full effect at around five weeks.

SAFETY CONCERNS

- Acupuncture generally is considered safe, provided a qualified, licensed practitioner uses sterilized, disposable needles.

- Make sure the practitioner uses a new set of needles from a sealed package. He or she should also swab the puncture site with alcohol before inserting the needle. If not performed properly, acupuncture can result in infection at the insertion site or organ puncture.

- Use a licensed practitioner

- Make sure your acupuncturist uses sterile, disposable needles

- Discuss using acupuncture with your medical doctor

- Tell your acupuncturist about any medication or supplements you are taking, or if you have a pacemaker, are pregnant or have breast implants

FINDING AN ACUPUNCTURIST

One of the best resources for locating a licensed acupuncturist may be your doctor – many physicians are familiar with the procedure and may make referrals. Several organizations also provide lists of acupuncturists:

- The American Academy of Medical Acupuncture
  Lists medical doctors who practice acupuncture.
  800-521-2262
  www.medicalacupunture.org

- The National Acupuncture and Oriental Medicine Alliance
  Lists state-licensed, registered
  or certified acupuncturists.
  253-851-6869
  www.acuall.org

- American Association of Oriental Medicine
Lists acupuncturists and Oriental medicine
practitioners by geographic area.
610-266-1433
www.aaom.org

Alexander Technique

Common uses:

Improve posture, reduce muscle tension

The Alexander technique teaches people how to properly move and align their bodies. The aim is to get rid of bad habits such as slouching or tensing parts of the body, allowing easier, freer movement.

The technique was developed by Frederick Matthias Alexander (1869-1955), an Austrian actor who feared losing his career when he began having bouts of hoarseness on stage. Alexander noticed that lowering his head and tensing his neck when he recited lines restricted his vocal chords. As he worked to change his posture, he found his voice improved. Other actors began to ask Alexander for help, and today many actors are taught the technique in performing arts schools.

The idea behind the technique is that proper alignment of the head, neck and spine is crucial to overall health. Improper alignment can cause muscles to tense and become painful. Once the head, neck and spine are correctly aligned, however, the rest of the body automatically will follow their lead, reducing muscle tension and making movement easier.

The Alexander technique is taught in groups or one-on-one settings. In both, an instructor observes the way students walk, sit, stand and bend and coaches students to relax neck muscles so the head balances freely on top of the neck. Using verbal instruction and gentle touch, the practitioner will show students how to improve posture during common activities, such as sitting at a desk. The number of lessons varies, and instructors usually suggest one-on-one coaching to customize the technique.

Because the chronic neck and back pain often associated with fibromyalgia can cause people to tense up their muscles, leading to more pain, the Alexander technique is sometimes recommended as a way to counter bad posture habits and reduce muscle pain.

SCIENTIFIC EVIDENCE

Clinical studies on the effectiveness of the Alexander technique are few and far between, and none have specifically addressed how the technique may benefit people with fibromyalgia. A 1999 study suggested the Alexander technique may help improve balance in healthy older women. [Jour Gerontol A Biol Sci Med Sci 1999 Jan; 54(1): M8-11] A 1996 study examined the effects of the Alexander technique in conjunction with other therapies, including acupuncture, chiropractic, education and psychological counseling, in 67 patients with back pain and found that this multidisciplinary approach reduced back pain. The effects were felt for six months after stopping therapy. [Clin Exp Rheumatol 1996 May-Jun; 14(3): 281]

SAFETY ISSUES

- The Alexander technique generally is considered safe for everyone, including pregnant women, when taught by a qualified instructor.

- If an instructor's suggestion about a different way to hold your body causes pain, stop.

FINDING A PRACTITIONER

The American Society of Teachers of the Alexander Technique certifies instructors who have completed at least three years of training and offers a referral service. To find an instructor or get more information on the technique, contact the organization at (800)473-0620 or on the Web at www.alexandertech.org.

Ayurvedic Medicine

Common uses:

To prevent or treat illness

Ayurveda, a comprehensive approach to health that originated more than 5,000 years ago in India, may be the oldest healing tradition in the world. Its name means "the science of life," and ayurveda is concerned with mental and spiritual health as well as physical well-being. It is still a main form of health care in India, where it is often used in conjunction with Western medicine.

The main principles of ayurveda involve balance, between the body, mind and spirit, and it concentrates on healthy living through diet, exercise, meditation, herbal and other therapies. Ayurveda focuses primarily on preventing illness, but an ayurvedic practitioner may also treat specific conditions. Each person is treated with a personalized, customized program that addresses specific symptoms.

Ayurveda holds that each person has a vital energy called *prana*, which is made up of a unique combination of five key elements – earth, air, fire, water and ether. These elements combine to form three types of *doshas*, or energies: *vata, pitta* and *kapha*. Each person has a unique proportion of the energies (with one dominating), and these energies are constantly shifting. Health is maintained by achieving balance between the energies.

Vata, or wind, is a combination of air and ether. Vata is associated with movement and controls circulation and breathing. A person in whom vata is dominant is said to be creative, quick-minded and restless, and they are thought to be prone to digestive problems.

Pitta, or bile, is made of fire and is the energy that governs digestion and metabolism. People in whom pitta is dominant are thought to be intelligent and competitive, and may be prone to fever and inflammatory diseases.

Kapha, or phlegm, is made of earth and water and governs the body's physical strength, immune system and structure. People in whom kapha is dominant are thought to be stable and grounded and are prone to colds and allergies.

When you visit an ayurvedic practitioner, he or she will examine you using a combination of techniques. For example, the practitioner will perform a physical exam, taking your pulse, looking at your tongue, eyes, fingernails and posture. The practitioner will also pay attention to non-physical symptoms, asking you about detailed questions about your lifestyle and listening to the tone of your voice. Based on this examination, the practitioner will identify your dominant energy and then develop a customized health plan that may include herbs, diet recommendations, massage, yoga, breathing exercises and purification techniques, or *panchakarma*, designed to eliminate toxins from the body. These techniques can include fasting, sweating and cleaning out the digestive tract by vomiting, using laxatives or enemas. These treatments usually are performed at special centers over the course of several days.

SCIENTIFIC EVIDENCE

Although there has been a great deal of interest in ayurvedic medicine, almost no scientific evidence exists to show whether or not it is effective. Because ayurveda stresses the mind-body connection, it can be a popular treatment for chronic conditions such as irritable bowel syndrome, chronic fatigue syndrome and fibromyalgia, conditions where both physical and psychological factors can influence symptoms.

One part of ayurvedic medicine – meditation – has been accepted by Western medicine as a way to reduce stress and promote overall well-being. Other forms of relaxation such as yoga and breathing exercises are also accepted as healthy practices. And many of its recommendations – eat a healthy diet that includes fresh fruits and vegetables, exercise regularly and take steps to reduce stress – are similar to what you might hear from a doctor of Western medicine.

Currently, researchers are examining whether ayurvedic medicine can be effective in treating cancer, high cholesterol, high blood pressure, diabetes and depression.

SAFETY CONCERNS

- Ayurvedic medicine is considered noninvasive, so there are few risks associated with it. Any combination of herbs should be evaluated by your medical doctor, because they might interact with conventional medicines.

- You should also tell your ayurvedic practitioner about any other drugs or herbs you are taking.

- Be sure to tell your medical doctor that you are using ayurvedic medicine, especially if any changes are recommended in your diet. If you have back or neck problems, talk with your medical doctor before performing yoga.

- Purification techniques that involve any equipment used inside your body may cause infection. Be sure the equipment is sterile. It's important to talk with your medical doctor before using any internal cleansing techniques.

FINDING A PRACTITIONER

Ayurvedic practitioners are not licensed in the U.S., which can make finding someone difficult. The ideal practitioner would be trained in both ayurvedic medicine and Western medicine. It's also more likely that insurance will cover your treatments if you see a doctor of Western medicine who also practices ayurvedic medicine.

Look for a graduate of Indian ayurvedic medical programs. He or she will have received a degree such as a bachelor of ayurvedic medicine or doctor of ayurvedic medicine and surgery from a qualified ayurvedic university in India.

The National Institute of Ayurvedic Medicine is the most comprehensive source of information on ayurvedic medicine in the U.S. Contact the organization by phone at (845) 278-8700 or on the Web at www.niam.com.

Balneotherapy

Balneotherapy involves bathing in warm water containing sulfur or other minerals or using mineral-rich mud baths. See hydrotherapy, page 162.

Belladonna

Common uses:
Treating headache, menopausal symptoms, irritable bowel syndrome, asthma, muscular pain

Belladonna is a toxic herb (also called deadly nightshade) that has been used for hundreds of years, both as a medicine and as a poison. Its name, "beautiful woman" in Italian, came about when women in the 16th century used the herb to dilate their pupils and flush their skin to appear more attractive.

Belladonna contains three toxic alkaloids, plant-based substances that contain nitrogen: scopolamine, atropine and hyoscyamine. An overdose of belladonna can be fatal. One of the alkaloids, atropine, is a central nervous system stimulant and is used to dilate pupils and as an antidote for nerve gas. Another, scopolamine, is used to treat motion sickness. Belladonna, combined with phenobarbital, is the ingredient in *Donnatal* and *Bellergal*, drugs used to treat irritable bowel syndrome, inflammation of the intestine, and ulcers, by reducing intestinal muscle spasms.

SCIENTIFIC EVIDENCE

Anticholinergic medications (which cause relaxation of the smooth muscles, such as the colon) have been used to treat irritable bowel syndrome for a number of years. Several studies were done in 1970s to examine belladonna's effect on irritable bowel syndrome; however, participants either received belladonna only in combination with phenobarbital or received only one of belladonna's alkaloids. [Br Med Jour 1979; 1 (6160):376 and Jour Clin Pharmacol 1978;18 (7):340] Most studies of belladonna have evaluated the herb in combination with other medications or in homeopathic dilutions. No scientific studies have looked at the effect of using belladonna alone to treat irritable bowel syndrome.

SIDE EFFECTS AND INTERACTIONS

Side effects are common and may include:

• Dryness of mouth, nose, throat or skin

- Constipation

- Flushing of the skin

- Dilated pupils

- Decreased sweating

- Drowsiness

- People with heart disease, gastrointestinal disease, glaucoma, Sjögren's syndrome or neuromuscular diseases, and pregnant or lactating women should avoid belladonna.

- Belladonna may affect the rate at which other drugs or supplements are absorbed, and may cause serious side effects if taken with any drugs that interact with anticholinergic medications, including tricyclic antidepressants and antihistamines.

SAFETY CONCERNS

- If you have an allergy or sensitivity to any plant in the nightshade family (common vegetables such as bell peppers, tomatoes, eggplants and potatoes), avoid using belladonna.

- Always check with your medical doctor or pharmacist before taking any product containing belladonna, and never give the herb to a child.

DOSAGE

Belladonna is extremely dangerous. There currently is no standardized preparation of belladonna, so the amount of alkaloids in any preparation may vary, meaning anyone who takes it risks a possible overdose. Because of the toxic nature of belladonna and danger of lethal overdose, the Food & Drug Administration warns consumers not to take this herb in any amount.

Biofeedback

Common uses:
Reduce pain, control body functions

Biofeedback combines technology and meditation techniques to help people learn to exert conscious control over body functions that are usually controlled by autonomic (unconscious) processes. It uses electronic sensors to record and display such things as skin temperature, muscle tension, brain waves, blood pressure and breathing rate. The measurements are displayed in a graph on a computer screen or by using a tone or light signal, and you learn to use meditation techniques to alter the physical effect you want to change (for example, relaxing your muscles).

After some practice, people who use biofeedback can pay attention to their body functions and modify them without using the electronic prompts.

During a biofeedback session, electronic sensors are attached to your body and then to a computer. The process is painless; the sensors are attached with glue or are fashioned to slip around your finger. A practitioner will guide you in mind-body techniques, such as deep breathing or visualization, to exert influence on your autonomic body processes. As you perform these techniques, the computer will show their effect on your body. The goal is for you to learn to recognize your body functions and use these techniques without the aid of the sensors. Each person learns these techniques at a different rate, so the number of sessions required varies.

SCIENTIFIC EVIDENCE

Several studies have shown that biofeedback can relieve pain and stress for a number of conditions, especially when used in conjunction with other relaxation and mind-body therapies. It has been used to improve function in people with high blood pressure, anxiety, migraines, chronic back pain and Raynaud's phenomenon. Several studies have found that people with fibromyalgia who learned biofeedback techniques report less pain, sleep better and show improvement in morning stiffness. [Jour Rheumatol 1987;14:820-5]

SAFETY CONCERNS

• Biofeedback is noninvasive and safe. There are no side effects, and once you've mastered the techniques you can use them to modify your body's responses anywhere.

FINDING A PRACTITIONER

Many medical doctors, physical therapists and psychologists use biofeedback. Your doctor may be a good source of referral to a biofeedback program, and your insurance may be more likely to cover the cost if your doctor makes a referral. Fees can range from $40 to $150 per session.

The Biofeedback Certification Institute of America certifies U.S. practitioners and provides referrals. For more information, contact the organization at (303) 420-2902 or on the Web at www.bcia.org.

Black Cohosh (Cimicifuga racemosa)

Common uses:
Treating menopausal symptoms, premenstrual syndrome, osteoarthritis, rheumatoid arthritis; anti-inflammatory to reduce muscle pain

Native Americans used black cohosh, an herb, for centuries to treat "female problems." Today it is often used to treat hot flashes associated with menopause. The name of this member of the buttercup family comes from the color of its root and from the Algonquin word for rough. It is also known as bugbane or black snakeroot, and was an ingredient in the most popular patent medicines of the 19th century.

The active ingredient of black cohosh is believed to be a chemical called 27-deoxyactein. The plant also contains phytoestrogens, plant compounds that work like estrogen in the body, and may contain small amounts of salicylic acid, an ingredient found in aspirin and some nonsteroidal anti-inflammatory drugs (NSAIDs).

SCIENTIFIC EVIDENCE
Several studies have suggested that black cohosh may help reduce the symptoms of menopause, but the studies

have been small and contained flaws in their design. [Ann Intern Med 2002 Nov 19; 137 (10): 805] Some experts think that black cohosh can alleviate menopausal symptoms without increasing the risk of breast cancer, but others disagree and more studies are needed to determine if the herb increases or reduces the risk of breast cancer.

Some research has indicated lack cohosh may reduce symptoms of osteoarthritis and rheumatoid arthritis, but the studies used a combination of herbs, so the effect of black cohosh by itself is not known. [Rheum Dis Clin North Am 2000; 26(1): 13]

Black cohosh has also been proposed as a pain reliever, but currently no studies exist to support that use. Some people make compresses of black cohosh tea to relieve muscle pain. Make the tea by boiling the herb's dried root in water for 20 to 30 minutes. Then, apply a compress that has been soaked in the tea to the painful area for about 20 minutes.

SIDE EFFECTS AND INTERACTIONS

- Black cohosh is usually well tolerated for up to six months. The most common side effect is mild stomach upset, which may be lessened by taking the herb with food.

- Based on animal studies and what is known about related plants, theoretical side effects could include headaches, low blood pressure and increased risk of osteoporosis.

- Black cohosh theoretically may increase the risk of bleeding and should not be used with other anticoagulants, such as heparin and warfarin (*Coumadin*); pain relievers, such as aspirin or NSAIDs; and herbs, such as ginkgo biloba and garlic.

• Due to its estrogen-like effect, black cohosh may increase the effects of supplements such as evening primrose oil and soy. It may also interfere with birth control pills or hormonal replacement therapy, and the breast cancer drug tamoxifen (*Nolvadex*).

• If you take medication for hypertension (high blood pressure), black cohosh may increase the drug's effect, lowering blood pressure even further.

SAFETY CONCERNS

• People with an allergy to aspirin or NSAIDs, or people with a seizure disorder, should avoid black cohosh.

• Pregnant and lactating women should not take black cohosh. The herb can cause premature labor.

• Because experts are not sure of the effect of its estrogen-like properties, women with a family history of breast or endometrial cancer should not take black cohosh.

• If you take black cohosh, be sure to tell your doctor and to stop before any surgery because of the risk of increased bleeding.

• Do not use black cohosh for more than six months.

DOSAGE

Doses of black cohosh frequently are based on the amount of 27-deoxyactein; a usual dose contains 1 mg to 2 mg of the chemical.

Boron

Common uses:

Treating osteoarthritis and osteoporosis; improving memory, hormonal regulation; helping the body metabolize magnesium

Boron is a trace mineral that helps the body use calcium and magnesium. Because it helps regulate how the body uses calcium, it may aid in preventing bone loss. The most common medicinal use of this mineral is in boric acid, often used as an eye wash. Boron is found in many fruits (apples, pears, grapes), vegetables, nuts and dried beans. Boron levels in food vary according to the amount of boron that was in the soil in which they were grown, but people who eat a diet rich in fruits and vegetables are likely to get enough boron.

SCIENTIFIC EVIDENCE

There is not a lot of scientific evidence to support the use of boron for most conditions, though one small study did suggest that boron may be useful in treating osteoarthritis. [Environ Health Perspect 1994 Nov; 102 Suppl 7:83] Also, research has noted that in some areas where the level of boron in the soil is low, there is a higher incidence of osteoarthritis. Most of its proposed uses stem from the way in interacts with calcium; for example, if boron helps the body retain calcium, then it may provide benefits in treating any condition that arises from calcium deficiency.

People with fibromyalgia sometimes use boron because it helps the body metabolize magnesium, which may reduce pain (see magnesium, p. 176). Boron deficiency is rare in the Unites States, and most people who eat a healthy diet get enough boron without taking a supplement.

SIDE EFFECTS AND INTERACTIONS

- A low dose of boron is usually well tolerated in adults, though some people may experience stomach upset and diarrhea.

- Other side effects may include irritation of the skin, mouth, eyes and throat.

- Large doses of boron can be poisonous.

- Boron may increase estrogen levels, which could raise the risk of cancer for some women, and should not be taken with birth control pills, hormonal replacement therapy or any drugs that contain estrogen.

- Boron may increase the level of calcium in the blood, especially if used with supplements that contain calcium.

SAFETY CONCERNS

- People with an allergy to boric acid, borax, citrate, aspartate or glycinate should avoid boron.

- Pregnant and lactating women should not take boron.

- Women with a family history of breast cancer or endometrial cancer should avoid boron, because it may increase estrogen levels in the body.

DOSAGE

There is no Recommended Daily Allowance for boron, but a dose of 3 mg to 6 mg has been used in studies. Because you may already get about 3 mg of boron from your diet and/or from a multivitamin, limit supplementation to under 3 mg per day. Boron is often combined with calcium in supplements, so make sure to check the labels.

Boswellia (Boswellia serrata)

Common uses:
Treating osteoarthritis, rheumatoid arthritis, asthma, inflammatory bowel diseases (Crohn's Disease, ulcerative colitis), bladder inflammation

The oil, resins and gum of Boswellia serrata, a tree from Asia, is also known as frankincense or salai guggal. It has been used in Indian ayurvedic medicine and Chinese medicine to treat arthritis, menstrual pain and as an external medication for bruises and sores. Some animal and test tube studies have shown that boswellia inhibits leukotriene synthesis, which contributes to inflammation. Historically, the herb has also been used as part of religious rituals and to enhance emotional well-being; and the oil from boswellia is found in food products and some cosmetics.

SCIENTIFIC EVIDENCE

There is some evidence to suggest that boswellia may be an effective treatment for asthma, [Eur Jour Med Res 1998;

3(11): 511] but not enough to prove it is effective for any other condition. Because the herb possesses anti-inflammatory properties, it has been suggested as a possible treatment for arthritis and inflammatory bowel disease. However, the studies that have been done were small or poorly designed, so it's not clear that boswellia provides any benefit.

One double-blind German study [Z Rheumatol 1998; 57(1):11] showed it had no effect on rheumatoid arthritis symptoms, but another that used boswellia in combination with other herbs showed participants got relief from pain and inflammation. The study [Indian Jour Pharm 1992; 24:98] combined boswellia with ginger, turmeric, ashwagandha (an Indian herb) and zinc. Because participants received other herbs, it is impossible to determine what effect boswellia had. Another study that sought to determine whether boswellia was effective in treating Crohn's disease seemed show those treated with the herb improved, but the study was poorly designed. [Z Gastroenterol 2001; 39(1):11]

SIDE EFFECTS AND INTERACTIONS

- Boswellia is usually well tolerated. The most common complaints in clinical trials were nausea and acid reflux; it may also cause diarrhea and a skin rash.

- Boswellia may increase the effects of cholesterol-lowering drugs and anticancer drugs. It may also decrease the effectiveness of nonsteroidal anti-inflammatory drugs such as ibuprofen (*Advil, Motrin, Nuprin*), aspirin and naproxen sodium (*Aleve*). Similar effects may occur with supplements, with boswellia increasing the effects of those used to treat joint disease (such as glucosamine and chondroitin), those that have anticancer properties, and those that lower cholesterol.

SAFETY CONCERNS

- Boswellia generally is considered safe and studies show it to be well tolerated with few side effects.

- Pregnant and lactating women should not take boswellia since there are reports in Indian literature of spontaneous abortion.

- Some experts think that use of boswellia in children can mask asthma symptoms, so make sure a medical doctor supervises any use.

DOSAGE

Various doses of boswellia have been studied, but it generally considered safe at 150 mg three times a day.

Bromelain (From pineapple, Ananas comosus)

Common uses:

Treating muscle aches, arthritis, heartburn; aiding digestion

Bromelain is a proteolytic (protein-digesting) enzyme found in pineapple. It is an anti-inflammatory and blood thinner, and works by breaking down fibrin, a blood-clotting protein. It also helps the body produce plasmin, a substance that blocks the production of inflammatory compounds. Bromelain supplements are made from enzymes found in pineapple stems and are one of the most popular supplements in the world.

SCIENTIFIC EVIDENCE

Because of its anti-inflammatory properties, bromelain often is used to treat sports-related injuries, such as sprains and strains, and seems to help bruises heal faster. A number of studies attest to bromelain's anti-inflammatory effect. A 1995 German open study, for example, found that people with strains and torn ligaments who took bromelain had a significant reduction in pain and swelling, comparable to people taking nonsteroidal anti-inflammatory drugs (NSAIDs). [Fortschr Med 1995 Jul 10; 113(19):303]

As a digestive aid, bromelain can boost the effect of digestive enzymes in the body such as trypsin or pepsin.

SIDE EFFECTS AND INTERACTIONS

- Bromelain has few side effects. Large doses can cause stomach upset or skin rash; people with ulcers should avoid taking bromelain.

- People who are allergic to pineapple should not take bromelain.

- Bromelain may increase the risk of bleeding when used with anticoagulants such as heparin or warfarin (*Coumadin*), or aspirin and other NSAIDs. The same applies to supplements that also increase the risk of bleeding, such as gingko biloba or garlic.

- Bromelain may increase the effects of tetracycline antibiotics.

SAFETY CONCERNS

- Bromelain generally is considered safe.

DOSAGE

Doses of enzymes are expressed in activity units or international units. Bromelain's effect is measured in GDUs (gelatin digesting units) or MCUs (milk clotting units). The amount of GDUs or MCUs in a milligram dose may vary. Common doses vary, too; some experts suggest 1,200 to 1,800 GDUs or MCUs per day, broken up into three doses, while other suggest doses as high as 3,000 GDUs or MCUs per day.

Take bromelain on an empty stomach for its anti-inflammatory properties; take it just before eating if you use it as a digestive aid.

Cat's Claw (Uncaria tomentosa, Uncaria guianensis)

Common uses:
Treating inflammation, boosting immune system, relieving chronic pain

Cat's claw is an herb derived from the inner bark of a woody vine that grows in the Amazon, mainly in Peru and Bolivia. Its name comes from the appearance of two curved thorns at the base of its leaves that look like cat's claws.

Although there are many related species, Uncaria tomentosa and Uncaria guianensis are harvested in the wild and used for treating various ailments. (There is also a plant native to the American Southwest, also called cat's claw, which is completely unrelated.) Look for these two kinds of cat's claw when buying supplements.

Cat's claw has been proposed as a treatment for many illnesses and conditions, including cancer, HIV, arthritis, irritable bowel syndrome, chronic fatigue syndrome and fibromyalgia. However, studies done so far have been inconclusive or are in early stages, and even natural medicine experts disagree on whether people with autoimmune diseases such as HIV should take cat's claw – some believe it helps the immune system, while others believe that it can make symptoms worse. In Germany and Austria, cat's claw is dispensed by prescription from medical doctors to improve immune-system response in cancer patients.

SCIENTIFIC EVIDENCE

Traditionally cat's claw has been used to relieve pain. Some test tube and animal studies suggest the herb may reduce inflammation, and may be useful in treating rheumatoid arthritis. The most promising study to date found that a daily dose of 100 grams of freeze-dried cat's claw reduced knee pain in people with osteoarthritis. [Inflamm Res 2001 Sep; 50(9):442]

SIDE EFFECTS AND INTERACTIONS

- Few side effects have been reported when using cat's claw at suggested doses. Possible side effects include stomach upset, nausea, headache and dizziness.

- Theoretically, cat's claw may increase the risk of bleeding when used with anticoagulants such as heparin or warfarin (*Coumadin*), or aspirin or nonsteroidal anti-inflammatory drugs. The same applies to supplements that also increase the risk of bleeding, such as ginkgo biloba or garlic – chamomile may add to the effect.

- There is some evidence that cat's claw may interfere with the way the liver breaks down some drugs and supplements, so if you use prescription drugs or any other supplements ask your medical doctor before taking cat's claw.

- Cat's claw may slow heartbeats or lower blood pressure, so don't use it if you are taking an antihypertensive medication or drugs to treat irregular heart rhythms.

SAFETY CONCERNS

- Cat's claw traditionally has been used as a contraceptive and to induce abortion, so pregnant women, women who are breast-feeding or those who wish to become pregnant should not take this herb.

- People with autoimmune disorders, such as rheumatoid arthritis, lupus, multiple sclerosis or HIV should avoid using cat's claw or use with caution, since it is not known whether the herb has a positive or negative effect on symptoms.

DOSAGE

Cat's claw is usually taken as a pill or a tea. A common dose is 250 mg taken twice a day. Cat's claw is also available as a tea, usually prepared as 1 teaspoon to 2 teaspoons of dried herb per cup, taken up to 3 times a day.

Cayenne (Capsicum)

Common uses:
Relieving pain, easing digestive upset

Cayenne, also known as chili pepper or hot red pepper, is a common ingredient in cooking hot, spicy dishes. Cayenne also has a reputation as a pain reliever and aid to digestion. Cayenne contains capsaicin, a substance that causes the body to release endorphins, natural painkillers.

Capsaicin is an irritating chemical that is also found in pepper sprays used for self-defense. Used topically in lower amounts, however, it eases pain by offering its own discomfort as a kind of diversion. It burns when first applied and possibly blocks pain signals by interfering with substance P, a chemical that transmits pain signals. Cayenne also is taken orally to aid digestion.

SCIENTIFIC EVIDENCE

Cayenne cream or ointment is recommended by the American College of Rheumatology as part of a treatment plan for osteoarthritis of the knee, and a pilot study suggests it may be effective in controlling muscle pain in fibromyalgia. [Semin Arth Rhem 1986;23(suppl 3):41]

Taken orally, cayenne may also aid digestion and help prevent ulcers by increasing blood flow in the stomach and intestines, by stimulating digestive juices, and by inhibiting growth of bacteria that may cause ulcers. Studies have shown that people who eat the highest level of hot peppers have the lowest incidence of peptic ulcers.

SIDE EFFECTS AND INTERACTIONS

- Cayenne has few side effects when used as directed; it does burn when first applied to the skin.

- If cayenne or capsaicin products come into contact with your eyes or mucus membranes, you may feel intense burning but no permanent damage. Be sure to wash your hands before touching your eyes after applying cayenne.

- At high doses, cayenne can cause diarrhea or stomach pain.

- Cayenne can be used or taken safely with drugs and other herbs.

SAFETY CONCERNS

- Don't use cayenne on broken or irritated skin.

- Keep cayenne away from children.

- Don't use cayenne on the same area where you use therapeutic heat, such as a heating pad or hot towel, as you increase a risk of burns.

DOSAGE

Use according to package instructions. A small, dime-sized amount of topical cream usually is effective for localized pain. When applying topically, leave cayenne on for about 30 minutes to give the capsaicin time to penetrate skin.

Ch-d

Chamomile (Matricaria recutita)

Common uses:

Treating insomnia, irritable bowel syndrome, heartburn, menstrual cramps, anxiety

Chamomile is one of the most popular herbs in the world and is often used to make a soothing tea, though it is also available in pill form. There are two types of chamomile – German chamomile (Matricaria recutita), which is the kind you'll find most often in the United States and the one that has been used in most studies, and English or Roman chamomile (chamaemelum), which is used mainly in England.

Though there is no scientific evidence that chamomile is an effective treatment for any health problem, the herb has long had a reputation for easing anxiety and helping digestion (when Peter Rabbit's mother put him to bed following his run-in with Mr. McGregor, she gave him a cup of chamomile tea). Chamomile appears generally safe for everyone, with few side effects.

SCIENTIFIC EVIDENCE

Chamomile has been investigated as a possible treatment for everything from the common cold to insomnia to digestive upset. It also is said to relieve rashes and help heal wounds.

Chamomile is believed to have a mildly sedating effect that may help people fall asleep easier. It also may relax the smooth muscles, helping digestion and easing menstrual cramps. As a sleep aid, the herb usually is taken as a tea before bedtime.

SIDE EFFECTS AND INTERACTIONS

- Chamomile is very well tolerated and side effects are rare. Extremely high doses may cause nausea and vomiting.

- Theoretically, chamomile may increase the risk of bleeding, so those using anticoagulants such as heparin or warfarin (*Coumadin*), or those taking aspirin or nonsteroidal anti-inflammatory drugs, should take care. The same applies to supplements that also increase the risk of bleeding, such as ginkgo biloba or garlic – chamomile may add to the effect.

- Chamomile may cause drowsiness and can increase the effect of drugs such as lorazepam (*Ativan*), phenobarbital, codeine and alcohol, as well as supplements such as valerian (see p. 225).

SAFETY CONCERNS

- People with allergies to the same plant family (asters, chrysanthemum, ragweed) should avoid chamomile.

- While chamomile is often said to be safe for pregnant and lactating women, it may in theory have an effect on the uterus, so it should be avoided during pregnancy.

- Because chamomile may cause drowsiness, use caution if you are driving.

- Do not take chamomile with alcohol.

DOSAGE

A common dose is 1 cup to 4 cups of chamomile tea daily (from tea bags) or 3 grams of fresh flower heads steeped in boiling water, taken 3 times a day. Most anecdotal evidence suggests chamomile is safe for children, at half the adult dose. However, consult your pediatrician before administering any herbal treatments to children.

Chinese Medicine

Common uses:
Preventing or treating illness, relieving pain

Traditional Chinese Medicine has been used for thousands of years and is widely practiced in Asia today, along with Western medicine. Acupuncture, massage and herbal medicine are the best known components of Chinese medicine in the U.S. Qi gong and tai chi (see p. 222), forms of exercise and moving meditation, are also part of Chinese medicine.

Underlying the principles of Chinese medicine is a belief in balance, expressed by two opposing but complementary forces, yin and yang. Yin and yang, sometimes called the feminine and masculine principles, are identified with certain organs in the body. Lungs, kidneys and the heart are associated with yin, and the stomach, intestines, bladder and gallbladder are associated with yang. For people to be healthy, yin and yang must be balanced. Various methods are employed to achieve this balance, including herbs and practices like acupuncture or exercise techniques.

Another concept is that of qi (see p. 222), which has no real English translation. Often called the life force, it is an invisible energy that flows through everything that is alive. It travels through the body in channels or meridians, and disease results when qi is blocked or out of balance. Treatments, then, are aimed at unblocking or strengthening the flow of qi.

To balance qi, a practitioner of Chinese medicine may suggest acupuncture, herbal medicines (most often in a formula that combines several herbs and supplements), and/or qi gong. Herbs are available in standard preparations, or the practitioner may mix a custom formula.

SCIENTIFIC EVIDENCE

Although there has been a great deal of interest in Chinese medicine, almost no scientific evidence exists to show whether or not it is effective. Because Chinese medicine emphasizes balance and disease prevention, it can be a popular treatment for chronic conditions such as irritable bowel syndrome, chronic fatigue syndrome and fibromyalgia.

Some aspects of Chinese medicine, such as acupuncture, have been studied and seem to be effective at lessening pain (see acupuncture, p. 79). Tai chi and qi gong have also been examined in a few Western studies, with promising results.

Some herbs may also help people with chronic conditions. A 1998 placebo-controlled study of people with irritable bowel syndrome found that those who received a standardized Chinese herb formulation or a customized formula showed significant improvements in symptoms versus the placebo group. [JAMA 1998 Nov 11; 280(18):1585-9]

When you visit a practitioner of Chinese medicine, he or she will examine you looking for a pattern of symptoms rather than an illness. The practitioner will perform a physical exam, visually examining your appearance, listening to your breathing and paying attention to your body odor and excretions, such as sweat or mucus. He or she will take your pulse in several places, examine your tongue, and ask detailed questions about your diet, sleep and elimination habits. Based on this examination, the practitioner will describe the diagnosis in terms of "qi deficiency" or blockage, and then develop a customized health plan that may include herbs, acupuncture, Chinese massage (stimulation of acupuncture points), diet advice and exercise techniques such as tai chi or qi gong.

SAFETY CONCERNS

- There are few safety concerns when a certified practitioner administers Chinese medicine. You should talk to your medical doctor before seeking Chinese medicine treatment.

- In acupuncture, make sure sterile, disposable needles are used.

- Use caution in taking herbal preparations. These formulas are not regulated as medicines, and some herbs from Asia may be contaminated with pollutants or heavy metals.

- Some herbs may interact with other supplements or drugs, or may have side effects. Consult your medical doctor.

FINDING A PRACTITIONER

Chinese medicine is not licensed in the U.S., so you may find a wide range of qualifications among practitioners.

The National Certification Commission for Acupuncture and Oriental Medicine certifies practitioners of acupuncture and Chinese herbalists. For a directory of certified practitioners, contact the organization at (703) 548-9004 or on the Web at www.nccaom.org. The Web site has a searchable database of practitioners.

Chiropractic

Common uses:

To treat back pain and some other pain conditions

Each year, some 20 million Americans see a chiropractor, making chiropractic the third-largest health-care profession in the country. Most people go to a chiropractor for neck or back pain following an injury. Chiropractic involves the manual adjustment or manipulation of the spine to relieve pain and restore normal movement.

Chiropractic began in 1895 when an Iowa man named Daniel David Palmer claimed to have restored the hearing of a nearly deaf man by adjusting his spine. Palmer believed that misalignments (called subluxations) of the vertebrae caused pinched nerves that were responsible for almost all diseases and illnesses. When the spinal column was properly aligned, the diseases would be cured.

For years, the American Medical Association (AMA) considered chiropractic to be quackery and encouraged medical doctors not to refer patients to chiropractors. In 1980, five chiropractors sued the AMA for restraint of trade and won. Now many health insurers cover chiropractic care, and some medical doctors refer patients with back pain to chiropractors.

While some chiropractors still adhere to the belief that manipulating the spine can treat everything from asthma to high blood pressure, many prefer to focus only on the treatment of back pain and are willing to have treatments evaluated by clinical studies. Some chiropractors also use alternative healing therapies, such as homeopathy and herbal medicine, or offer massage and acupuncture.

At your first visit, the chiropractor will take your medical history and perform a physical exam to rule out any conditions that should not be treated with chiropractic care. He or she may also order X-rays. You will be asked to remove just enough of your clothing so the chiropractor can manipulate your spine (or, if you wear loose clothing, you may not have to remove anything). He or she will move your joints, searching for those that are out of line.

Spinal manipulation generally is done barehanded, but the chiropractor may also use a machine or instrument to apply pressure. He or she will press a joint into place or gently ease it into alignment. You may feel some discomfort, but it should not be painful. If you hear a sound, it's not your joint cracking; the sound is just air moving around within the joint during adjustment.

SCIENTIFIC EVIDENCE

There is no evidence that chiropractic can treat a wide variety of diseases. Scientific evidence for the effectiveness of chiropractic care for back pain is mixed. In 1994, the federal Agency for Health Care Policy and Research reviewed more than 4,000 studies on low back pain and concluded that manipulation of the spine seemed to provide temporary relief in acute cases. The agency noted that such therapy appeared effective only when used as a short-term treatment.

A more recent study, however, suggested that chiropractic was no better at relieving back pain than physical therapy and only a little better than reading an educational booklet on back care. [N Engl Jour Med 1998 Oct 8; 339(15):1021] Chiropractors have challenged the study's design and procedures.

A pilot study that examined 21 people with fibromyalgia suggested that four weeks of spinal and soft-tissue manipulation and stretches improved range of motion and lessened pain. [Jour Manipulative Physiol Ther 1997 Jul-Aug; 20(6): 389] Another small study, not rigorously controlled, found similar results using spinal manipulation and ischemic compression (pressure applied on trigger points). [Jour Manipulative Physiol Ther 2000 May; 23(4):225]

SAFETY CONCERNS

- Chiropractic generally is considered safe for simple back pain. However, people with rheumatoid arthritis or osteoarthritis, sciatica (leg pain caused by nerve damage or pressure), osteoporosis or severe back pain that interferes with daily activities should see their medical doctor before visiting a chiropractor. A reputable chiropractor will not offer spinal manipulations for these conditions.

- There is no evidence to indicate that chiropractic can treat anything other than back pain. Some research suggests that chiropractic manipulation of the upper spine (neck area) may temporarily lessen neck pain, but experts say to be cautious – this kind of manipulation can further harm an already damaged spinal cord.

- Tell your chiropractor about your fibromyalgia and any medicines, herbs or supplements you take. In particular, using anticoagulants or supplements that have an anticoagulant effect (such as ginger or ginkgo) can increase the risk of bruising or bleeding.

- A chiropractor may take X-rays on your initial visit, but repeat X-rays are not necessary.

- Stop treatment immediately if your symptoms get worse, or if you don't improve after one month of treatment.

FINDING A CHIROPRACTOR

Chiropractors are trained in four-year schools of chiropractic and licensed in all 50 states. Ask your medical doctor to recommend a chiropractor, or contact the organization below.

American Chiropractic Association
(800) 986-4636
www.amerchiro.org

Chlorella (Chlorella pyrenoidosa)

Common uses:
Anti-oxidant, boosting immune system

Chlorella is a single-celled, green alga that is grown commercially, purified and made into a powder. Like its relative, spirulina, it is packed with proteins, vitamins and minerals and is rich in chlorophyll and beta-carotene, two substances with anti-oxidant properties. In fact, chlorella has the highest concentration of chlorophyll of any plant. Chlorella growth factor (CGF), a water-soluble extract, contains amino acids, nucleic acids and peptides, as well as vitamins and proteins.

SCIENTIFIC EVIDENCE
Research in Japan has suggested that chlorella stimulates growth and wound healing, boosts the immune system and may help prevent cancer. Two recent studies specifically examining the effects of chlorella on fibromyalgia indicated that taking a daily dose of chlorella may help relieve symptoms and improve quality of life. [Jour Musculoskel Pain; 2001:9(4):37] Another study [Altern Ther Health Med 2001 May-Jun; 7(3):79] examined chlorella to see whether consuming natural foods packed with macronutrients had any effect on people who otherwise eat a non-vegetarian diet; participants included people with fibromyalgia, high blood pressure and ulcerative colitis. Chlorella appeared to improve symptoms, though more research is needed.

SIDE EFFECTS AND INTERACTIONS

- Chlorella has no known side effects.

- Chlorella may contain vitamin K, which can counteract the effect of warfarin (*Coumadin*). People taking this drug should talk to their medical doctor before taking chlorella.

SAFETY CONCERNS

- No safety concerns have been noted with chlorella.

- Dosage

- Suggested doses range from 300 mg to 1,500 mg per day.

Coenzyme Q10 (Ubiquinone)

Common uses:

Treating fibromyalgia; preventing heart disease, congestive heart failure, gum disease, Alzheimer's disease, Parkinson's disease, cancer

Discovered in the 1950s, coenzyme Q10 is a natural substance found in every cell of the body as well as in all animal and plant life. Indeed, its scientific name, ubiquinone, comes from the word ubiquitous. Coenzyme Q10 acts as a catalyst to help cells produce energy from food. It works with enzymes (hence the name coenzyme) to speed up the metabolic process and provide energy needed for healthy muscles. It has become one of the most popular supplements in the world.

Coenzyme Q10 is most abundant in the cells of the heart, and much of the research on the supplement has focused on its use for heart disease. Some people with fibromyalgia take coenzyme Q10 to boost energy and to repair muscles, though there is no definitive scientific evidence yet of these effects.

Coenzyme Q10 has also been touted as an anti-aging supplement, because amounts of the compound decrease as people age, and as an anti-oxidant.

SCIENTIFIC EVIDENCE

Some studies have shown that coenzyme Q10 is effective in combination with other prescription medications for treating congestive heart failure, after heart attacks, lowering blood pressure, relieving angina and protecting against heart attacks.

Studies pertaining to fibromyalgia have been mixed. It has been suggested that one of the problems contributing to fibromyalgia is that people with the condition do not produce enough adenosine triphosphate (ATP), which the body uses for fuel. Although theoretically a deficiency of coenzyme Q10 could contribute to the lack of ATP, a 1998 study found no difference in the levels of coenzyme Q10 in the muscles and blood of people with fibromyalgia and a control group of healthy people. [Clin Exp Rheumatol 1998;16:513]

However, an open-label, uncontrolled study [Jour Int Med Res 2002 Mar-Apr;30(2):195] evaluated the effects of coenzyme Q10 combined with ginkgo biloba on quality of life in people with fibromyalgia, and found that after 84 days, 64 percent of participants said they felt better. A controlled study is now planned.

When purchasing coenzyme Q10, look for gel-caps or tablets that have the compound in an oil base; it is better absorbed that way.

SIDE EFFECTS AND INTERACTIONS

- Coenzyme Q10 has very few side effects.

- Some people using coenzyme Q10 may experience stomach discomfort or nausea, headache, difficulty sleeping or flu-like symptoms.

- People taking anticoagulants such as heparin or warfarin (*Coumadin*) should not take coenzyme Q10 without consulting their medical doctor; in theory, the compound may increase the risk of bleeding.

- People taking supplements with a similar effect, such as ginkgo biloba or garlic, should use caution.

- Coenzyme Q10 may increase the risk of blood clots, so people with clotting disorders should also talk to their doctors before taking the compound.

- Vitamin E may increase the effects of coenzyme Q10.

SAFETY CONCERNS

- Except for the drug interactions noted above, coenzyme Q10 generally is considered safe.

- Pregnant and nursing women, and people with heart disease, should check with their medical doctor before taking coenzyme Q10.

DOSAGE

There are no established doses, and various studies have used different amounts of the compound. However, coenzyme Q10 does not appear to be dangerous even in large doses. A typical dose might be 50 mg twice a day. One of the drawbacks to using coenzyme Q10 is its cost; a daily dose of 100 mg can cost about $40 per month.

Devil's Claw (Harpagophytum procumbens)

Common uses:

Anti-inflammatory; relieving pain, digestive problems

The name devil's claw comes from the many small hooks that cover this plant's fruit, designed to cling to animals in order to spread its seeds. Native to Africa, devil's claw has long been used to treat digestive problems and arthritis. The root, the part of the plant used for medicinal purposes, contains harpagoside, which has anti-inflammatory and painkilling properties.

SCIENTIFIC EVIDENCE

Devil's claw is promoted as a pain reliever for fibromyalgia. Scientific evidence is mixed: An animal study showed that devil's claw did not reduce swelling even at high doses. [Can Med Assoc Jour 1983 Aug 1; 129(3): 249] However, another study indicated that people with arthritis who take devil's claw might be able to reduce their use of NSAIDs. [Joint Bone Spine 2000; 67(5): 462] Another study suggested that devil's claw reduced low back pain significantly better than placebo. [Phytomedicine 2002 Apr;9(3):181]

SIDE EFFECTS AND INTERACTIONS

- Devil's claw has relatively few side effects. The most common are diarrhea and gastrointestinal irritation.

- Devil's claw may increase the amount of stomach acid, so people with ulcers should not use the herb.

- Devil's claw should not be taken with antacids, H2 antagonists such as cimetidine (*Tagamet*), famotidine (*Pepcid*) and ranitidine (*Zantac*), or proton pump inhibitors such as lansoprazole (*Prevacid*) and omeprazole (*Prilosec*).

- Devil's claw may decrease blood sugar levels, so people taking oral medication or insulin for diabetes should not take devil's claw without first talking to their medical doctor.

- Devil's claw may increase the risk of bleeding when used with anticoagulants such as warfarin (*Coumadin*) or heparin, and NSAIDs such as aspirin, ibuprofen or naproxen sodium. Similar effects may occur with herbs that have anticoagulant properties, such as ginkgo biloba and garlic.

SAFETY CONCERNS

- Devil's claw generally is considered safe.

- Pregnant and breast-feeding women should avoid devil's claw, as it may stimulate contractions.

DOSAGE

A recommended dose is 50 mg to 100 mg of standardized harpagoside daily, taken on an empty stomach.

DHEA (Dehydroepiandrosterone)

Common uses:

Treating Addison's disease, menopause, lupus, rheumatoid arthritis, lack of energy

DHEA is a mild androgen, or male hormone, that is produced in the body by the adrenal glands. DHEA is converted into testosterone and estrogen. It has been promoted as a supplement that can slow aging, prevent osteoporosis, treat cancer, aid in weight loss and increase sex drive. However, current evidence doesn't support most of these claims. So far, DHEA has shown some promise in treating lupus, Addison's disease (adrenal insufficiency) and some symptoms of menopause.

Both men and women make DHEA, and levels decline significantly with age. At age 60, for example, our bodies make just 15 percent as much as when we were 20. Because the body produces less DHEA as it ages, it has been suggested that DHEA can prevent some age-related problems, specifically heart disease in older men. Researchers are investigating this possibility.

Contrary to popular opinion, wild yam does not contain DHEA.

SCIENTIFIC EVIDENCE

One theory suggests that DHEA is useful in treating fibromyalgia because the symptoms are a result of chronic stress on the adrenal glands, and people with fibromyalgia sometimes have lower levels of DHEA in their blood. According to this theory, taking DHEA will boost energy levels. However, no studies have been done using DHEA as a treatment for fibromyalgia.

SIDE EFFECTS AND INTERACTIONS

- Few side effects have been noted when DHEA is taken at recommended levels. The most common side effects are headache, fatigue and nasal congestion.

- Because DHEA is used to make estrogen and testosterone, some side effects are similar to those caused by these hormones. At larger doses, for example, women may develop acne, facial hair, deepening of the voice and mood swings, and men may experience increased blood pressure, aggression and breast tenderness. Theoretically, DHEA may increase the risk of breast, ovarian or prostate cancer.

- DHEA may raise blood sugar levels, so people with diabetes should not take DHEA unless supervised by their medical doctor.

- Women who take DHEA may lower their levels of HDL (good cholesterol).

- DHEA may change the way the liver breaks down some drugs, such as triazolam (*Halcion*), causing the levels of these drugs to become too high. Taking

DHEA with azathioprine (*Imuran*) or methotrexate can result in liver damage.

- In theory, DHEA may increase the risk of blood clots.

- Drugs such as alprazolam (*Xanax*) may increase the levels of DHEA in the body, which could cause an increase in side effects.

SAFETY CONCERNS

- Only take DHEA under a doctor's supervision. Because healthy people under age 50 do not need DHEA supplementation, you should first talk to your doctor and have a blood test to determine the level of this hormone in your body. Only if your level is low should you consider taking DHEA. DHEA should only be taken to raise hormone levels to a normal range, not to exceed it, so it is critical for your doctor to monitor the levels in your blood.

- Have your doctor check for any hormone-related cancers (such as breast cancer and prostate cancer) before you take DHEA.

- Women who are pregnant or breast-feeding should not take DHEA. Do not give DHEA to children.

- Remember, DHEA is not a "natural" supplement—it is manufactured chemically, and it is stronger than many herbs or nutrients. The safety of its long-term use is not known.

DOSAGE

A maximum dose of DHEA should not exceed 25 mg a day for men, and as little as 5 to 10 mg a week can often maintain normal levels in the blood.

Ephedra, Ma huang (Ephedra sinica)

Common uses:
Treating asthma; aiding weight loss; treating fatigue or lack of energy

Ephedra, also called ma huang in Chinese medicine, comes from dried stems of a shrub that grows in Asia. Its primary active ingredients are the chemicals ephedrine and pseudoephedrine, both stimulants that act on the central nervous system. In fact, ephedra's effect is similar to that of amphetamines ("uppers" or "speed") or adrenaline.

Ephedra increases the heart rate, raises blood pressure, speeds up the metabolism and functions as a diuretic. Traditionally used as a bronchodilator to treat asthma, ephedra is found in some supplements promoted for use by people with fibromyalgia to give an energy boost.

Ephedrine has been associated with at least 22 deaths, and the U.S. Food and Drug Administration has mandated all products containing ephedrine have a label stating possible adverse affects, that they contain no more than 8 mg of ephedrine per serving and be used for no more than seven days.

SCIENTIFIC EVIDENCE

Although ephedra was used for years to treat asthma, more modern drugs have been developed that are much safer. Ephedra has been touted as a weight-loss supplement (often combined with caffeine), and some studies suggest it may be effective [Int J Obes Relat Metab Disord 2002 May; 26(5):593]. Many of these studies have some problems in their design, however, and show contradictory results. Ephedrine has also been used to control blood pressure in women who have received spinal anesthesia during delivery.

Although ephedra is effective in treating some conditions, such as asthma, it is not considered safe. In addition, given the role that sleep disturbances may play in fibromyalgia, people with the condition should avoid ephedra's stimulant effects, which can cause insomnia.

SIDE EFFECTS AND INTERACTIONS

- Ephedra's side effects can be very dangerous. They include diarrhea, vomiting, anorexia, constipation and increased urine production, and possible liver damage.

- Ephedra may cause dizziness, irritability, restlessness, anxiety, euphoria, fainting and difficulty sleeping. Extremely serious side effects such as seizures and stroke can also occur.

- Ephedra can also affect the heart and lungs, causing breathing difficulties or irregular heartbeats. It can raise blood pressure, so those with this high blood pressure or heart disease, and those taking MAO inhibitors for depression, should avoid ephedra.

- Ephedra also interacts with a number of drugs and supplements, so anyone taking the supplement should discuss possible dangerous interactions with their medical doctor. Central nervous stimulants, theophylline and caffeine increase the stimulant effect of ephedra. The combination of ephedra and caffeine may even be fatal.

• Ephedra may lower blood sugar levels, and may increase the effects of insulin or oral drugs taken for diabetes, or supplements such as bitter melon.

• Pregnant and breast-feeding women should not take ephedra, nor should it ever be given to a child.

SAFETY CONCERNS

• The long list of safety concerns and the potential of fatal side effects associated with ephedra make this supplement a poor choice for anyone to take.

• If you do take ephedra, monitor your heart rate (pulse) and blood pressure. If your heart rate seems faster than normal or your blood pressure rises, stop taking ephedra.

DOSAGE

While ephedra-containing products usually list dosages on their packaging, there are serious risks associated with ephedra use. In February 2003, the Department of Health and Human Services announced that dietary supplements containing ephedra "may present a significant and unreasonable risk of illness and injury." Therefore, it is probably wise to avoid using ephedra at all.

Evening Primrose Oil (Oenothera biennis)

Common uses:

Treating skin conditions, rheumatoid arthritis, diabetes, breast pain or cysts, premenstrual syndrome; Raynaud's phenomenon; inflammation

Oil from the seeds of the evening primrose plant contains gamma-linolenic acid (GLA), which is one of the two main kinds of essential fatty acids. GLA is an omega-6 fatty acid; the other type is omega-3 (see entry under fish oil). The body converts GLA into prostaglandins and leukotrienes, which can affect pain and inflammation. GLA may help the body produce anti-inflammatory prostaglandins.

Although the body generally makes all the GLA it needs from foods containing linolenic acid, no one food has a tremendous amount of GLA. Evening primrose oil is one source; however, borage oil contains even more GLA.

Some experts recommend taking an evening primrose supplement that contains vitamin E, since the fatty acids in evening primrose oil break down rapidly and vitamin E slows the process. Not all the omega-6 fatty acids in evening primrose oil wind up as GLA – some can be converted into arachidonic acid, which is used to make the prostaglandins and leukotrienes that cause inflammation.

SCIENTIFIC EVIDENCE

Evening primrose oil is widely used in Europe to treat diabetic neuropathy (nerve damage) and eczema, a common skin rash. Early research indicates it may indeed help reduce nerve pain caused by diabetes [Diabet Med 1990 May;7 (4):319]. The evidence for using evening primrose oil in treating eczema is mixed, and no studies have indicated that it actually helps reduce symptoms of Raynaud's phenomenon.

Evening primrose oil appears to lessen the breast tenderness some women experience prior to their periods, but the studies done so far lacked significant controls and data, so better studies are needed. Studies done to see whether evening primrose oil is effective in treating PMS have been severely flawed, so no conclusion has been reached.

Several small studies have suggested that very high doses of GLA may help reduce joint swelling and tenderness in people with rheumatoid arthritis. [Ann Pharmacother 1993;27:1475]

No studies have been done specifically examining the effects of evening primrose oil on fibromyalgia. Evening primrose oil is promoted as a supplement for people with fibromyalgia as an anti-inflammatory and for pain relief.

SIDE EFFECTS AND INTERACTIONS

- Evening primrose oil generally has few side effects. Sometimes people experience bloating or stomach upset, side effects which can be lessened by taking the supplement with food.

- There is a risk of seizure when evening primrose oil is used with anesthesia, so you should stop taking it before any surgery.

- Evening primrose oil also has an anticoagulant effect, and may increase the risk of bleeding when used with other anticoagulants such as heparin or warfarin (*Coumadin*), or aspirin or NSAIDs. The same applies to supplements that also increase the risk of bleeding, such as ginkgo biloba or garlic.

- Evening primrose oil should not be taken with drugs to lower blood pressure.

- People who have epilepsy or those taking anti-seizure medications should not take evening primrose oil.

SAFETY CONCERNS

- Evening primrose oil generally is considered safe.

DOSAGE

Doses range from 240 mg of GLA a day to 1,800 mg. Be sure to check the label to see how much GLA the supplement contains – look for high dosage capsules to avoid taking a handful several times a day. A safe dose for pregnant and breast-feeding women has not been established.

Feldenkrais Method

Common uses:

To improve posture, reduce muscle tension

The Feldenkrais method is used as a way to become more aware of your body – how it moves and how you hold various positions. Developed by Moshe Feldenkrais (1904-1984), a Russian physicist, after a knee injury, the Feldenkrais method is somewhat difficult to describe, because it depends on the interaction between you and your instructor. Basically, this "body re-education" encourages you to be aware of your bones, muscles and joints and teaches you to recognize bad habits in posture and movement that may cause you to tense up and stress other parts of your body. Without that tension, you can gain expanded range of motion and flexibility.

The Feldenkrais method emphasizes an inner awareness of the body and movement, so that actual changes in the way one moves are tied to a self-image of movement and intention. Popular with dancers and musicians who regularly perform repetitive movements, this program is sometimes recommended by doctors or physical therapists, since the movements are gentle and not painful. People with fibromyalgia may try this method before beginning an exercise program, because it can help them learn proper movement and lessen the chances of injury.

The Feldenkrais method is taught in classes and one-on-one; students may use either training option or both. In Awareness Through Movement classes, taught in groups, the instructor guides students through gently movements using common body positions, with the aim of improving in a classroom, students explore basic movement themes to improve movement awareness and function. Often the class will focus on one movement theme, with verbal instructions from the teacher. These classes usually meet once a week for four to six weeks.

One-on-one instruction is offered in Functional Integration lessons. Using a slow and gentle touch, the instructor guides the student's body through a series of movements. The instructor uses touch to communicate and guide, not to correct, and there is no massage-like pressure applied. Instead, the instructor tries to make the student aware of habitual patterns of movement and suggests new ways to move. The number of individual sessions depends on the student and the teacher.

SCIENTIFIC EVIDENCE

Few studies have been done specifically examining the effect of this method on fibromyalgia. One pilot study evaluated the effect of the method compared to a pool exercise program for people with fibromyalgia and found that although improvements in balance and better muscle function in the legs occurred in the Feldenkrais group, they were not sustained. [Jour Musculoskeletal Pain, 2001; 9(4): 25]

SAFETY CONCERNS

- The Feldenkrais method generally is considered to be quite safe. Make sure you find a qualified instructor and tell him or her about any physical limitations.

- Pay attention to your body, and stop if you move in a way that hurts.

- The Feldenkrais method does require a commitment of several weeks to attend classes and apply the techniques learned.

FINDING AN INSTRUCTOR

Look for an instructor certified by the Feldenkrais Guild of North America, the professional organization for the method. Contact the guild at (800) 775-2118 or on the Web at www.feldenkrais.com for a list of practitioners in your area. Some physical therapists and other health-care practitioners become guild-certified.

G-h

GABA (Gamma-aminobutyric acid)

Common uses:

Treating insomnia, anxiety, epilepsy

Gamma-aminobutyric acid, sometimes called the body's "natural tranquilizer," is an amino acid neurotransmitter that helps reduce stress-related nerve impulses. It may promote relaxation and sleep, and it is thought that people with insomnia, anxiety and epilepsy may not produce enough GABA.

Many anti-anxiety drugs, such as diazepam (*Valium*), and some herbs such as valerian, work by targeting GABA receptors in the brain to induce relaxation and sleep, so it is thought that increasing levels of GABA by taking supplements of the chemical itself may also help. However, GABA has barely been studied in humans and there is little information about its effectiveness or safety.

SCIENTIFIC EVIDENCE

GABA manufactured by the body does not cross the blood-brain barrier very well, so it seems doubtful that taking GABA orally would have much effect. One study suggested a high intake of GABA produced elevated levels of plasma growth hormone and prolactin, but more studies are needed to determine GABA's effect. [Acta Endocrinol (Copenh) 1980 Feb; 93(2):149]

Although GABA has been proposed as a treatment for epilepsy – due to the fact that standard epilepsy drugs increase levels of GABA in the brain – studies have not shown the supplement to have any effect on epilepsy.

SIDE EFFECTS AND INTERACTIONS

- The side effects of GABA are unknown, because it has not been studied sufficiently in humans.

- Larger than usual doses may cause increased anxiety, nausea, numbness around the mouth and tingling in the arms and legs.

- GABA may increase the side effects caused by drugs that affect GABA receptors in the brain. Do not combine GABA with benzodiazepines such as diazepam (*Valium*), temazepam (*Restoril*) and lorazepam (*Ativan*).

- Valerian may also affect GABA receptors, so you should not combine GABA with valerian.

SAFETY CONCERNS

- Not enough is known about GABA to determine if it is safe.

DOSAGE

Because of the lack of information, suggested doses vary. One suggested dose for insomnia is 500 mg at bedtime.

Ginger (Zingiber officinale)

Common uses:

Easing nausea, joint pain and muscle pain

Ginger is used widely as a spice, but the herb also has medicinal properties and is most often used to settle an upset stomach. Ginger enhances digestive fluids and neutralizes acids in the stomach. Early American settlers drank ginger beer, an ancestor of ginger ale, for that purpose. Although most commercial ginger ales today have only miniscule amounts of ginger, natural ginger ales do contain enough of the herb for therapeutic effect. Ginger is one of the mostly widely used natural treatments for a variety of ailments, and fresh ginger root can be found in almost any supermarket today. Ginger is also available in supplement form for easier use as a treatment.

Laboratory research also indicates ginger is an anti-oxidant and anti-inflammatory, and may reduce pain by inhibiting the production of prostaglandins and leukotrienes, which cause pain and swelling.

SCIENTIFIC EVIDENCE

Several studies have examined ginger's nausea-relieving properties. Results have been mixed: There is some evidence that ginger is effective in treating motion sickness, and nausea caused by other drugs or anesthesia. [Br J Anaesth 2000;84 (3):367] Ginger has also been studied to see if it helped women with severe nausea during pregnancy; several small studies suggested it was indeed effective.

An uncontrolled study of the effect of ginger on arthritis and muscle pain showed that all patients with musculoskeletal pain found relief, and three-fourths of those with rheumatoid arthritis or osteoarthritis also saw a decrease in pain and swelling [Med Hypotheses 1992 Dec; 39(4):342]. Ginger has also been used along with boswellia, turmeric and ashwagandha in similar study with similar results.

Most people with fibromyalgia who take ginger do so for its digestive benefits and to reduce muscle pain.

SIDE EFFECTS AND INTERACTIONS

- Ginger generally has few side effects; the most common is occasional heartburn. At very high doses ginger may irritate the lining of the stomach.

- Ginger may increase the risk of bleeding when used with anticoagulants such as warfarin (*Coumadin*) or heparin, or NSAIDs.

- Similar effects may occur with herbs that have anticoagulant properties, such as ginkgo biloba and garlic.

- In theory ginger may increase the drowsiness caused by some drugs, including benzodiazepines such as lorazepam (*Ativan*), barbiturates such as phenobarbital, narcotics and alcohol, and herbs such as valerian.

- People who take insulin or oral drugs for diabetes should be monitored by their medical doctor when taking ginger, because the herb may lower blood sugar levels.

SAFETY CONCERNS

- Ginger is considered safe.

- Though ginger has been studied for morning sickness, pregnant or breast-feeding women should not take ginger without discussing it with their medical doctor first.

- You may need to stop taking ginger before any surgery, because of the risk of increased bleeding.

DOSAGE

Doses range according to therapeutic intent. A common dose is 1 g to 4 g per day or fresh powdered ginger or 100 mg to 200 mg of standard extract in pill form. Fresh or freeze-dried ginger may be more effective. A 1/4 to 1/2 inch slice of ginger root is roughly equal to the common dose. You can drink it steeped in water as a cup of tea or simply increase the amount of ginger you use in cooking.

Ginkgo Biloba (Ginkgo biloba)

Common uses:
Treating Alzheimer's disease, dementia, cerebral vascular disease, depression, Raynaud's phenomenon; age-related memory loss; poor circulation; "fibro fog"

Ginkgo biloba is a tree that can live as long as a thousand years. The tree sometimes is referred to as a living fossil, because the species has been on the earth for more than 200 million years. The herb is extracted from the leaves of the tree.

Ginkgo biloba extract is one of the most popular herbs in the world. It increases the flow of blood to the brain and central nervous system, and may have anti-oxidant properties. Contained in gingko biloba extract are flavone glycosides (organic substances that have anti-oxidant properties) and terpene lactones (chemicals called ginkgolides and bilobalides that improve blood flow).

Use supplements that contain ginkgo biloba extract, or GBE. Take only standardized extracts. Look for products containing 24 percent flavone glycosides and 6 percent terpene lactones. It usually takes four to six weeks, and even up to 12 weeks, before you notice any effect.

SCIENTIFIC EVIDENCE

Some double-blind studies have indicated that gingko biloba extract can either produce some positive effect on or delay deterioration of mental function in people with age-related dementia including Alzheimer's. The herb appears to be most effective in the early stages of Alzheimer's, and the effects are modest. [Neuropsychobiology 2002;45(1):19] Ginkgo may also help relieve depression and anxiety in older people.

People with fibromyalgia sometimes take ginkgo to relieve fatigue, improve concentration and combat "fibro fog." Although ginkgo often is promoted as a memory aid, there is mixed evidence that it helps improve memory in healthy people of any age. A double-blind German study in 2000 found that a combination of gingko and ginseng did improve cognitive function in healthy volunteers. [Psychopharmacology

(Berl) 2000 Nov;152(4):353] Other studies using ginkgo alone [JAMA 2002 Aug 21;288(7):835] have shown no effect.

Because ginkgo improves blood flow to the arms and legs, it has been proposed as a treatment for Raynaud's phenomenon. A controlled German study showed it increased blood flow in finger capillaries [Arzneimittelforschung 1990 May;40(5):589], so it may help with symptoms of Raynaud's.

Ginkgo is being studied as a possible treatment to speed up recovery from stroke and to treat circulatory and nervous system conditions, because of its ability to increase blood flow.

SIDE EFFECTS AND INTERACTIONS

- Ginkgo has few side effects; a mild headache or stomach upset is possible.

- In rare cases, it may cause nausea, restlessness or irritability, although these effects are usually mild and go away.

- Ginkgo may increase the risk of bleeding when used with anticoagulants such as heparin or warfarin (*Coumadin*), or aspirin and other NSAIDs. The same applies to supplements that also increase the risk of bleeding, such as ginger or garlic.

- Because of the increased risk of bleeding, you should stop taking ginkgo before surgery.

SAFETY CONCERNS

- Ginkgo generally is considered safe for long-term use.

- Ginkgo's effects on pregnant and breast-feeding women are not known, so it should be avoided during that time.

- Never use unprocessed ginkgo leaves to make a tea – they contain a possible neurotoxin.

DOSAGE

A common dose of ginkgo biloba extract is 40 mg to 80 mg two or three times a day.

Ginseng (Panax)

Common uses:

Treating fatigue, stress, diabetes, high blood pressure, impotence and male infertility; improving cognitive function; liver protection

There are several types of ginseng, an herb that has been used for centuries to reduce fatigue, boost sex drive and fight cancer. Asian ginseng (Panax ginseng) is the kind used in most supplements. American ginseng (Panax quinquefolius) is grown mainly in the Midwest and exported to China. Siberian ginseng (Eleutherococcus sinticosus) is a related herb that claims to have many of the same properties, but has not been studied as extensively.

The part of the plant used for medicinal purposes is the root, which is usually harvested after four to six years, when its active ingredients, called ginsenosides, are at their peak. Old, wild roots are considered the most valuable, while cultivated rootlets are viewed as lesser quality. Ginseng is processed in two forms – "white" is the dried root, while "red" has been steamed and dried. Because older roots harvested in the wild are rare, ginseng is expensive – up to $20 per ounce.

SCIENTIFIC EVIDENCE

Ginseng may help fight a number of illnesses. Animal research and a small number of human studies have shown that it stimulates specialized immune cells called "killer T cells" that help rid the body of infections. Some studies have suggested it may have cancer-fighting properties, but the studies have been small and not well designed. [Nutr Rev 1996 Nov; 54(11 Pt 2): S71]

There is conflicting evidence about whether ginseng helps mental function. A number of studies have suggested that ginseng can improve mental processing and attention in healthy people, [Hum Psychopharmacol 2002 Jan; 17 (1): 35] but other studies have shown no effect. [Eur J Clin Pharmacol 1999 Oct; 55(8): 567]

Likewise, studies have suggested that ginseng may lessen fatigue and reduce stress by acting as a central nervous system stimulant, but the evidence is not conclusive.

SIDE EFFECTS AND INTERACTIONS

- Ginseng has few side effects at recommended doses.

- Some people may experience nervousness, stomach upset, insomnia, or headache. The combination of ginseng and caffeine can increase these side effects.

- Higher doses of ginseng may affect a woman's menstrual cycle or cause breast tenderness.

- Ginseng may affect blood clotting and may increase the risk of bleeding when used with anticoagulants such as heparin or warfarin (*Coumadin*), or aspirin and other NSAIDs. The same applies to supplements that also increase the risk of bleeding, such as gingko biloba or garlic.

- Because of the increased risk of bleeding, you should stop taking ginseng before surgery.

- Ginseng may interfere with how the liver breaks down some drugs and may cause the level of drugs in the body to be too high or too low.

- Ginseng can also affect the level of herbs and supplements in the body. Ask your doctor before taking ginseng if you are taking any prescription drugs or other supplements.

- Ginseng may lower blood sugar levels, so people taking insulin or oral medications for diabetes should consult their medical doctor to ensure their blood sugar levels are closely monitored before taking ginseng.

- Do not take ginseng if you also take MAO inhibitors.

SAFETY CONCERNS

- Ginseng generally is considered safe.

- It is not known whether ginseng can cause birth defects, so pregnant and breast-feeding women should not take the herb.

DOSAGE

There is no standard dose for ginseng; it depends on the ginsenoside content. Look for a product that is standardized to 7 percent ginsenoside. For pills and capsules, a dose of about 100 mg twice a day has been used; for powdered root, about 500 mg to 1,000 mg per day. Some experts recommend you stop taking ginseng for a week after you have used it for two or three weeks.

Grape Seed Extract (Vitis vinifera, Vitis coignetiae)

Common uses:
Anti-oxidant; promoting cardiovascular health; preventing vision problems, slowing retinopathy

Grape seed extract is a flavonoid, a plant substance with anti-oxidant properties that protect cells from damage by free radicals (unstable oxygen molecules). As its name suggests, the extract is made from the seeds, and sometimes the skins, of red grapes.

Some laboratory tests suggest that active ingredients in grape seed extract, called procyanidolic oligomers (PCOs) or proanthocyanidins, have 50 times greater anti-oxidant activity than Vitamin C or E. PCOs may also improve blood circulation and help strengthen blood vessels, and may help reduce swelling after surgery or injury.

People with fibromyalgia may take grape seed extract because its anti-oxidant power may help protect muscle cells from damage.

SCIENTIFIC EVIDENCE

Some studies indicate that people who consume higher levels of flavonoids have a lower risk of heart disease. [Am Jour Clin Nutr 2002 Sep; 76(3):560 and Am Jour Epidemiol 1999 May 15;149(10):943], so it's possible that the PCOs in grape seed extract offer protection against heart disease. Whether that is actually the case, however, has not been established – other studies show no benefit. [Am Jour Epidemiol 1999 May 15;149(10):943] Animal studies have indicated that PCOs may lower blood cholesterol levels and protect against arterial plaque formation, and may improve circulation.

Several small studies also indicate grape seed extract can slow the progression of retinopathy (retinal damage caused by diabetes or high blood pressure) by improving circulation in the tiny blood vessels of the eye. [Bord Med 1978;11:1467]

SIDE EFFECTS AND INTERACTIONS

- Grape seed extract has very few side effects. Some people may experience headache, dizziness, nausea or a dry, itchy scalp.

- Theoretically, grape seed extract may increase the risk of bleeding when used with anticoagulants such as heparin or warfarin (*Coumadin*), or aspirin and other NSAIDs. Grape seed extract theoretically may also increase the anticoagulant action of other supplements such as gingko biloba or garlic.

- Because of the increased risk of bleeding, you should stop taking grape seed extract before surgery.

- Grape seed extract may increase the effectiveness of vitamins C and E.

SAFETY CONCERNS

- Grape seed extract generally is considered safe.
- Pregnant and breast-feeding women should not take the herb without talking to their medical doctor first.

DOSAGE

A common dose of grape seed extract is 100 mg to 300 mg daily. Look for supplements that are standardized to contain 92 percent to 95 percent PCOs. Because only about 30 percent of the PCOs from grape seed extract remain in your body 24 hours after ingestion, you need to take grape seed extract regularly to have any benefit.

Green tea (Camellia sinensis)

Common uses:
Treating arthritis, cancer prevention, anti-aging; anti-oxidant

Green tea contains potent anti-oxidant chemicals called polyphenols that have been shown to reduce inflammation and protect against cancer. Green tea has been used medicinally in Asia for hundreds of years, and population studies suggest that green tea consumption may be one reason why cancer rates are lower in Japan. Green tea may also protect against heart disease by lowering cholesterol and blood pressure, promote longevity, prevent tooth decay (green tea contains fluoride), and help heal gum infections.

Both black tea and green tea are derived from the same plant, but they are processed in different ways. Green tea is made by steaming the leaves, while black tea is oxidized; oxidation of black tea prevents the polyphenols from having any therapeutic use or benefit.

SCIENTIFIC EVIDENCE

Although green tea is known to be a potent source of anti-oxidants, much of the research into its benefits has taken place in test tube and animal studies in the laboratory. One study in China found that people who drank as little as one cup of green tea a week for six months reduced their risk of developing some kinds of cancers (rectal, pancreatic and others) than did people who drank less or no green tea.

It is thought that green tea's anti-oxidant properties may prevent or reduce the symptoms of osteoarthritis. This claim has not been fully substantiated. One animal study showed that mice given extracts of green tea polyphenols had a lower rate of arthritis than mice which did not receive the extract, and those that did develop arthritis had only mild cases. [Proc Natl Acad Sci USA. 1999 Apr 13;96 (8):4524]

Green tea contains caffeine, which may cause side effects for some people taking green tea regularly as a therapy. Some teas and supplements are available in decaffeinated form, but it is not known whether they are as effective as a treatment.

Side Effects and Interactions

- Most side effects of green tea come from its caffeine content. Caffeine can cause nervousness, sleeplessness or anxiety in some people. Caffeine is also a diuretic.

- A cup of brewed tea has about 40 mg of caffeine, but some supplements contain less (about 5-6 mg in two 250 mg pills).

- Side effects can include irritability, sleeplessness, irregular heartbeat, dizziness, vomiting, diarrhea, headache and loss of appetite.

- Caffeine can increase the side effects of certain drugs, including tricyclic anti-depressant drugs and theophylline, and supplements such as ephedra.

Safety Concerns

- Green tea is considered safe. However, people with fibromyalgia need to consider whether the benefits of green tea outweigh the possible sleep problems caused by caffeine. You could opt for a decaffeinated version, but researchers aren't sure whether you would get the same anti-oxidant benefits.

- Look for a pill form of green tea that doesn't contain as much caffeine as the brewed tea, and take it early in the day.

- Because of the caffeine content, pregnant and breast-feeding women should not consume green tea.

- Do not consume more than 250 mg of caffeine per day.

DOSAGE

A typical dose of green tea is about three cups a day, containing about 240 mg to 320 mg of polyphenols, or about 100 mg to 300 mg in pill form.

Guaifenesin

Common uses:

Treating fibromyalgia

Guaifenesin is a treatment for fibromyalgia that has received a lot of attention among people with the disease, and sparks controversy among many doctors and other experts. The compound originally came from a tree bark extract called guaiacum and was used to treat arthritis in the 1500s. Now it is synthesized in a laboratory and is a common ingredient in cough syrups and cold medicines (used as an expectorant, it thins mucus in the lungs).

Guaifenesin, or "guai," was proposed as a treatment for fibromyalgia by Paul St. Armand, MD, who theorized that people with fibromyalgia have a defect in their kidneys that allows phosphates to build up in the body. The excess phosphates are stored in the bones, muscles and tendons, interfering with the body's ability to produce ATP, which it uses for energy. Eventually, "lumps and bumps" form in the muscles. Guaifenesin is supposed to help the kidneys excrete phosphates, preventing the buildup in the body and reducing the symptoms of fibromyalgia.

However, there is no scientific evidence to indicate that guaifenesin does anything for fibromyalgia. While the supplement isn't dangerous, the rules people who take guaifenesin must follow result in an increase in symptoms that may affect quality of life and well-being.

The "guai protocol," the name for the regimen of guaifenesin treatment proposed by Dr. St. Armand and others, is extremely demanding. Patients must have the lumps and bumps "mapped" by a medical doctor to determine the proper dosage, and avoid concentrated salicylates, chemicals found in all plants and concentrated in some medications (such as aspirin), topical ointments, supplements and cosmetics, including some deodorants, toothpastes, mouthwashes and makeup. Even proponents warn that a worsening of symptoms is to be expected for the first several months of treatment and that patients may "cycle," or experience periodic flares that can be very painful.

The urine and sweat of people taking guaifenesin will become dark and smelly. Proponents say that these symptoms are a sign the protocol is working and the body is excreting built-up phosphates.

Currently, high doses of guaifenesin are available only by prescription. Proponents of the guaifenesin protocol urge people with fibromyalgia to attempt the treatment only under the care of a medical doctor.

SCIENTIFIC EVIDENCE

The sole clinical study of guaifenesin showed that the substance had no effect on the symptoms of fibromyalgia. In 1996, Robert Bennett, MD, and Dr. St. Armand collaborated on a double-blind study where 20 women with fibromyalgia took 600 mg of guaifenesin twice a day and another 20 took a placebo twice a day. All were instructed to avoid salicylates. Participants were evaluated for blood and urinary levels of uric acid and phosphate, tender points, and other symptoms of fibromyalgia. At the end of the study, there was no difference between the group taking guaifenesin and the group taking a placebo.

Proponents of guaifenesin and the protocol (including Dr. St. Armand) claimed the study was unintentionally flawed because researchers did not know about salicylate levels found in cosmetics and participants continued to use them. However, Dr. Bennett holds that if the salicylates found in cosmetics affected the treatment, blood and urinary tests would have indicated that.

SIDE EFFECTS AND INTERACTIONS

- Guaifenesin, when used to thin mucus (as a treatment for respiratory illnesses), generally is considered safe.

- Nausea and vomiting are the most common side effects.

- People who take guaifenesin for fibromyalgia can expect a worsening of their symptoms for the first several months of treatment and periodic flares thereafter. Proponents claim it takes about two months to rid the body of a year's accumulation of phosphates.

• Proponents of the guaifenesin protocol claim salicylates counteract ("block") the treatment's effectiveness. People who take guaifenesin for fibromyalgia must avoid all contact with salicylates, even skin contact.

• Some people who follow the guaifenesin regimen say hypoglycemia (low blood sugar) can interfere with treatment. Proponents recommend a low-carbohydrate diet for people with hypoglycemia.

SAFETY CONCERNS

• Guaifenesin generally is considered safe.

• Pregnant and breast-feeding women should avoid guaifenesin, as its safety in those cases is not known.

DOSAGE

Proponents of the guaifenesin protocol suggest doses of 300 mg to 600 mg twice a day, under the care of a medical doctor.

Guided Imagery

Common uses:
Reducing pain, stress

Guided imagery harnesses the power of your imagination to help alleviate pain and anxiety, boost your self-image and maintain your body's well-being. You consciously use your mind to create images of health and well-being, which can help you relax, improve your immune system and reduce pain.

Guided imagery and visualization are often used inter-changeably; both use visual images in the mind to enhance health. The main difference is that guided imagery involves using a practitioner or an audiotape to lead you through the process of creating mental pictures.

Practitioners believe that guided imagery works because the brain perceives the mental image as actual experience. In other words, if you picture yourself relaxing on a beach somewhere, your brain is likely to tell your muscles to relax and to slow your pulse, lower your blood pressure and release endorphins, the body's natural painkillers.

While some medical doctors are skeptical how much influ-ence guided imagery has on an illness, it is an accepted prac-tice in Western mainstream medicine that is used to reduce pain, overcome addictions, lessen stress and treat phobias.

Although books on guided imagery are available, you may want to start by working with a practitioner or buying an audiotape (alternatively, you can tape your own guided imagery script). With a practitioner, it should take just a few sessions to master the technique, and the practitioner may allow you to tape the session to use at home.

Guided imagery sessions may start with a practitioner asking you questions about places that make you feel happy, favorite vacation or childhood spots, activities you love, etc. Next, the practitioner will lead you through a relaxation or breathing exercise, then guide you through a visualization exercise involving all five of your senses, perhaps suggesting specific images and sensations or asking you to choose images that have meaning for you. The specific type of exercise depends on what you want to accomplish: For example, you may imagine yourself free of pain or doing an activity you love. Or you may imagine your body fighting off symptoms of fibromyalgia, or watching those symptoms melt away.

With practice, you will be able to call up these healing images anywhere and at any time to promote relaxation and pain relief.

SCIENTIFIC EVIDENCE

Most scientific studies examine visualization in concert with other mind-body techniques such as relaxation, and there is no evidence that visualization actually helps cure disease. In promoting relaxation, however, it reduces stress and improves quality of life, and can make a difference in diseases and conditions where stress is a significant factor.

A number of studies have suggested that visualization can relieve pain. [Cancer Nurs 1997 Apr;20(2):79] One study that specifically examined the effects of guided imagery and amitriptyline (*Elavil*) on people with fibromyalgia found that participants instructed in "pleasant imagery" did better on pain scores than either a control group or a group which practiced attention imagery on the "active workings of the internal pain control systems." Participants were also randomly assigned *Elavil* or placebo, with neither showing any effect. [Jour Psychiatr Res 2002 May-Jun;36(3):179]

SIDE EFFECTS AND INTERACTIONS

- Guided imagery and visualization have no side effects.

- People with mental illness, especially those who experience hallucinations, should talk in advance with a trained therapist.

- You may wish to talk with a mental-health professional if you experience disturbing images or memories due to guided imagery.

SAFETY CONCERNS

- Guided imagery and visualization are considered safe for everyone.

- Be sure to focus on positive images.

- Let the practitioner know if any images are disturbing to you.

FINDING A PRACTITIONER

Practitioners of guided imagery are not certified or licensed, but the techniques are taught by many mental-health professionals. The best way to find a practitioner is to ask your medical doctor for a referral, or ask friends whom you trust. Check out the practitioner's references. Many hospitals and wellness centers also offer classes.

If you want to learn guided imagery on your own, audiotapes that help you visualize are often available at bookstores.

The Academy for Guided Imagery maintains a referral list of practitioners. Contact the organization at (800) 726-2070 or on the Web at www.interactiveimagery.com.

Hydrotherapy

Common uses:
Reducing pain, stiffness, inflammation

Hydrotherapy is simply the use of water (hold and cold treatments) to treat disease and injury. Ice, steam, and hot, tepid and cold water are all used in a variety of different ways, from baths and whirlpools to wraps and packs. Hydrotherapy is an element of physical therapy at almost every hospital and medical center. Exercises in hydrotherapy pools, whirlpool baths and swimming pools are often used for rehabilitation.

Hydrotherapy makes use of the way the body reacts to hot and cold, and to the pressure exerted by water on the skin. Cold decreases the body's activity, constricting blood vessels and numbing nerves, while heat increases circulation and dilates blood vessels. A hot bath may help relax tense muscles, while an ice pack can help reduce inflammation. In a whirlpool, the moving water has a massage-like effect on your body. Whirlpools, also known as spa baths or Jacuzzi tubs, are excellent treatments for many types of muscle pain and arthritis.

Contrast hydrotherapies alternate the application of heat and cold and are mainly used to stimulate circulation in a part of the body. A 30-minute bath alternating heat and cold (four minutes hot, one minute cold) can produce a 90 percent increase in blood flow.

The easiest and most common form of hydrotherapy is a hot bath. Some people with fibromyalgia find that a hot bath can ease sore muscles (people with myofascial pain, however, may find that it aggravates their symptoms) or that a bath before bedtime helps them sleep better. You may choose to add oils or herbs to the bath to help you relax. You can read, meditate or listen to music while soaking in a bath. Keep the water no hotter than 110 degrees Fahrenheit and don't stay in the bath for more than 15 minutes.

Cold or ice application can help ease pain, particularly after exercise. Place ice in a plastic bag, or use a bag of frozen vegetables, wrap it in a towel and apply to the painful area for 20 minutes. Wait 20 minutes before applying again.

Balneotherapy is a form of hydrotherapy that involves water that is rich in minerals such as sulfur. In addition, there are balneotherapy treatments that involve soaking sore limbs or the whole body in special, mineral-rich mud baths or soaks.

SCIENTIFIC EVIDENCE

Heat and cold treatments, and hot baths, are accepted forms of treatment for minor sprains, aches and muscle pains. One study examining balneotherapy at a Dead Sea spa found that people with fibromyalgia who took sulfur baths had improved physical functioning compared to a control group, and the benefits lasted up to three months. [Rheumatol Int 2001 Apr; 20(3):105]

SAFETY CONCERNS

- Hot immersion baths, whirlpool spas and saunas are not recommended for people with diabetes, women who are pregnant, or people with high or low blood pressure.

- Don't use a microwave to heat a compress – it can get too hot quickly. Instead, soak it in hot water.

- Don't apply ice directly to the skin – wrap it in a towel.

- Do not combine heat or cold treatments with topical counter-irritants such as capsaicin; you may incur a risk of burns.

- If you are pregnant or have heart disease, talk to your doctor before taking a sauna.

- People with Raynaud's phenomenon should avoid cold application.

Hypnotherapy

Common uses:

Relieving pain, anxiety, fear; treating irritable bowel syndrome; addressing behavioral issues such as smoking or diet

Hypnotherapy, or hypnosis, is a kind of deep relaxation and focused awareness. It has been used for centuries, but modern hypnotism began in the late 18th century when an Austrian doctor named Franz Anton Mesmer began treating people with magnets. Although that therapy was exposed as a fraud, Mesmer's success with it was due to his ability to soothe and persuade people – to "mesmerize" them.

Hypnosis is used today to bring about changes in behavior and thinking, and a hypnotic state can result in lower blood pressure, decreased heart rate and slower brain activity. Contrary to what you see in the movies, hypnosis can't be used to make you do anything you don't want to do. Basically, it is a state of altered consciousness that allows you to concentrate intently, making the use of visualization, relaxation or mind-body techniques more productive. Some people learn to hypnotize themselves, and a hypnotherapist can teach you the techniques to use.

In a hypnotherapy session, you will be guided through a relaxation exercise by a practitioner who uses a slow and soothing tone of voice. When you are deeply relaxed, you will still be aware of your surroundings but you will be more open to suggestion. Those suggestions depend on the goals you have for the therapy – you may focus on relieving pain, for example. The depth of your trance depends on many factors, including your willingness to undergo hypnosis and your own imagination. During a hypnosis session, you may feel both profoundly alert and relaxed at the same time.

SCIENTIFIC EVIDENCE

Hypnotherapy has been used alone or in combination with other therapies to control bleeding and reduce nausea after surgery; to control morning sickness and shorten labor in pregnant women, to stop smoking or overeating, and to treat stomach ulcers, skin conditions and abnormal heart rhythms.

Studies have also indicated that hypnotherapy can relieve the symptoms of irritable bowel syndrome, sometimes fully. In 1995, a National Institutes of Health panel recommended that hypnotherapy be considered part of the medical treatment for chronic pain.

In a randomized, controlled study that specifically targeted fibromyalgia, researchers found that a group of people who underwent hypnosis had a greater decrease in pain, fatigue and other symptoms than a group who underwent physical therapy. [Jour Rheumatol 1991 Jan;18(1):72]

Scientists aren't sure exactly how hypnosis works to relieve pain, but positron emission tomography (PET) scans of the brain show that certain areas of the brain affecting both sensation and emotion are activated by a painful stimulus. One of these areas, called the anterior cingulate cortex (ACC), seems to have an impact on how much pain is experienced. Other PET scans have shown that hypnosis affects the ACC, possibly reducing the sensation of pain.

SAFETY CONCERNS

- Hypnosis has little risk of side effects. It does not work for everyone. Using a professional hypnotherapist will incur a cost; be wary of excessive charges or any professional who tries to convince you to continue hypnosis at length if you do not see results.

FINDING A PRACTITIONER

Hypnotists are not licensed or regulated, so search carefully for a practitioner. The organizations below provide referrals of certified hypnotists.

National Guild of Hypnotists
(603) 429-9438
www.ngh.net

American Council of Hypnotist Examiners
(818) 242-1159

I-|

Kava (Piper methysticum)

Common uses:
Treating anxiety, pain; muscle relaxant; sleep aid

The kava (also known as kava kava) plant in a member of the pepper family that grows in the Pacific Islands and Hawaii, where is has long been used as a drink for social occasions and religious ceremonies. Its Latin name means "intoxicating pepper" and it has a tranquilizing effect that lessens anxiety without dulling the mind. It is not considered to be addictive. Alternative names for kava in various products containing the herb include kew, kawa-kawa, rauschpfeffer, sakau, tonga, wurzelstock and yangona.

The part of the plant used for medicinal purposes is the root, which contains active compounds known as kavalectones. Researchers aren't sure how kava works but believe it may affect the limbic system, a primitive part of the brain that controls emotions, among other functions.

Although doctors in Europe had long prescribed kava as a tranquilizer, recent reports of liver damage, some severe enough to require organ transplants, have led Germany, Switzerland and Great Britain to ban over-the-counter sales of kava. In the U.S., the Food and Drug Administration has issued a warning about kava. Some herbalists believe careful use of kava at recommended doses for short periods of time is not dangerous, but others advise avoiding the herb entirely.

Scientific Evidence

A number of clinical studies have shown that kava is an effective treatment for anxiety. [Jour Clin Psychopharmacol 200;20(1):84] Kava has not been studied specifically for fibromyalgia, but it is thought to be a muscle relaxant that may help reduce muscle spasms and lessen muscle pain. In addition, kava is used as a sleep aid.

Side Effects and Interactions

- Until recently, kava was thought to be safe when used at suggested doses for up to two months. However, there are reports of liver toxicity and death among kava users occurring even at doses previously thought safe.

- Signs of liver toxicity include increased fatigue, nausea, yellow skin, dark urine, yellowing of the eyes, and light-colored stools.

- The most common side effect is an upset stomach. Long-term use may cause dry, scaly, yellow skin.

- Kava can increase the drowsiness caused by drugs that affect the central nervous system, such as antidepressants, tranquilizers, sedatives and alcohol, or herbs such as valerian. Kava may also increase the effects of MAO inhibitors and of some herbs that may act like MAO inhibitors (such as evening primrose oil).

- Kava may enhance the effects of anesthesia and should not be taken two to three weeks before surgery.

- Kava should not be used if you are taking any medication that affects the liver, including acetaminophen (*Tylenol*).

SAFETY CONCERNS

- Because of the potential for liver damage, kava is best avoided.

- If you do take kava, do so only under the supervision of a medical doctor, who can monitor liver function. Do not take kava at higher than the recommended dose for more than one month.

- Avoid kava if you have a liver disease, such as hepatitis or cirrhosis.

- People with Parkinson's disease should not take kava – the herb can aggravate symptoms.

- Pregnant and breast-feeding women should not take kava.

- If you experience any side effects related to liver toxicity, stop immediately.

DOSAGE

Kava has dangerous risks associated with its use, so this supplement should be avoided.

Lavender (Lavendula angustifolia)

Common uses:

Treating anxiety, sleeplessness, pain, digestive problems

Lavender, a flowering, evergreen shrub that is native to the Mediterranean, has a long history of use. The Romans used it to scent their baths. Lavender aromatherapy is believed to be relaxing; many soaps and perfumes use lavender scent. Oil of lavender is used in Europe, both topically and internally, to treat everything from sunburn and minor scrapes to anxiety. Lavender tea is used in Germany to treat stomach upset and gas.

SCIENTIFIC EVIDENCE

There is some evidence that lavender aromatherapy may help relieve anxiety and promote relaxation. [Jour Adv Nurs 1995 Jan; 21(1):34 and Int Jour Neurosci 1998;96(3-4):217] A small study of people with rheumatoid arthritis showed mixed results. After using massage with lavender aromatherapy, most reported no pain relief; however, participants used fewer painkillers after the study, so they may have felt less pain. But it's not clear whether the benefit, if any, came from massage or aromatherapy. [Nurs Stand 1998;13:34]

An ingredient in lavender, perillyl alcohol, is being studied for the treatment of various cancers (breast, pancreatic, intestine); and animal studies at the University of Wisconsin at Madison found that rats given this extract showed a reversal in growth of advanced mammary tumors, and human clinical trials are underway. [Clin Cancer Res 2000;6(2):390]

SIDE EFFECTS AND INTERACTIONS

- As aromatherapy, lavender has few side effects.

- Lavender may cause a skin rash after contact.

- Some people report nausea, headache and chills after inhaling lavender.

- Large doses of perillyl alcohol taken internally can cause constipation, drowsiness and confusion.

- Taken by mouth, lavender may increase the amount of drowsiness caused by some drugs, including benzodiazepines such as diazepam (*Valium*), temazepam (*Restoril*) and lorazepam (*Ativan*); barbiturates; narcotics; antidepressants such as fluoxetine (*Prozac*); antihistamines; or alcohol. Lavender may also increase the side effects of some herbs, such as valerian, chamomile or kava.

- Taken by mouth, lavender may increase the risk of bleeding when used with anticoagulants such as warfarin (*Coumadin*) or heparin, and NSAIDs such as aspirin, ibuprofen or naproxen sodium. Similar effects may occur with herbs that have anticoagulant properties, such as ginkgo biloba and garlic.

- In theory, lavender taken by mouth may increase the cholesterol-lowering properties of other drugs and supplements.

SAFETY CONCERNS

- Lavender aromatherapy is considered safe.

- Pregnant and breast-feeding women should avoid taking lavender by mouth.

- Lavender should be used internally with caution, because of potential side effects. Talk to your doctor.

DOSAGE

For aromatherapy, add five to seven drops of essential oil of lavender to bath water, or two to four drops to three cups of boiling water and inhale the steam. Only use dried flowers to make tea; never use oil. Add one to two teaspoons of dried lavender flowers to one cup of hot water.

Magnesium

Common uses:

Treating cardiovascular disease, fibromyalgia, kidney stones, high blood pressure, premenstrual syndrome, diabetes

The mineral magnesium is essential to any number of functions in the body. It is involved in producing ATP for energy, relaxing muscles, and the formation of bones and teeth. It also helps the body produce and use insulin and helps regulate heart rhythm. It's not uncommon for Americans to be deficient in magnesium, because of a diet that is heavy in processed foods. Alcohol, some diuretics, antacids, birth control pills, estrogen, zinc, potassium and manganese can all reduce the level of magnesium in the body.

Due to its muscle-relaxing properties and its role in helping the body make ATP, magnesium has shown promise as a treatment for fibromyalgia, often combined with malic acid (extracted from apples), a substance that enhances the absorption of magnesium and may also play a role in helping the body make ATP. Many medical doctors recommend this combination for people with fibromyalgia. Magnesium is often combined with calcium, as well; high doses of magnesium diminish the effects of calcium in the body and vice versa, so many supplements have a balanced dose of both.

Magnesium supplements can contain a variety of types of magnesium. Look for a brand that has magnesium citrate, as it is most easily absorbed by the body. Some experts recommend taking vitamin B6 along with magnesium.

SCIENTIFIC EVIDENCE

A few well-designed clinical trials have looked at the effects of magnesium supplementation on fibromyalgia. Some studies have shown that people with fibromyalgia have low levels of magnesium or of ATP.

A 1995 placebo-controlled study examined the effect of magnesium and malic acid on people with fibromyalgia and found that high doses relieved pain and boosted energy. [Jour Rheumatology 1995;22(5):953] Another placebo-controlled study found similar results combining magnesium with malate; participants taking the supplement saw improvement within 48 hours. [Jour Nutr Med 1992;3:49]

SIDE EFFECTS AND INTERACTIONS

• Magnesium generally has few side effects. The most common are diarrhea and nausea. Because of the tendency for magnesium to lead to increased bowel movements, some doctors recommend it to patients that have constipation (especially due to use of certain types of drugs like tricylic agents).

• Extremely high doses (more than 6 grams per day) can be toxic, but such overdoses are rare.

• Several drugs interact with magnesium. Many diuretics, oral contraceptives and estrogen-replacement therapy can deplete magnesium in the body. Magnesium may interfere with the absorption of antibiotics in the tetracycline and quinolone families, digoxin, antacids, and bone-building drugs such as alendronate (*Fosamax*), etidronate (*Didronel*) and risedronate (*Actonel*). Do not take magnesium within two hours of these drugs.

- Magnesium also interacts with certain blood-pressure medications. Talk to your doctor before taking magnesium if you take any drugs for blood pressure.

- Magnesium can cause blood sugar levels to drop when used with some oral diabetes drugs.

- Magnesium also interacts with several minerals, including calcium and potassium. A high calcium intake combined with a high vitamin D intake (from dairy foods) can decrease absorption of magnesium. Vitamin B6 increases the absorption of magnesium.

SAFETY CONCERNS

- Magnesium generally is considered safe. People with kidney disease should not take magnesium, because their bodies may not be able to eliminate excess magnesium.

- People taking prescription medications of any kind should talk with their medical doctor before taking magnesium to check for interactions.

- If diarrhea develops after taking magnesium supplements, reduce the dose you are taking or take magnesium gluconate or magnesium sulfate. Both of these supplements are easier to digest.

DOSAGE

A recommended dose for fibromyalgia is 500 mg to 1,000 mg, combined with 1,200 mg to 2,400 mg of malic acid, divided into several doses and taken daily. Take magnesium with food, unless you eat a high-fiber diet. In that case, take between meals.

Magnetic Therapy

Common uses:
Relieving pain

The belief that magnets can help healing is an old one. The ancient Greeks used lodestones (natural magnets) as a therapy for various problems. In the sixteenth century, Swiss alchemist and physician Philippus von Hohenheim (known as Paracelsus) supposedly used magnets to treat illness. Magnets are now popular as a treatment to reduce the pain of arthritis, fibromyalgia, muscle strains, back pain and other types of pain.

No one is sure how magnets work to relieve pain. Some believe magnetic fields can penetrate the body and affect individual cells or organs. Various theories have suggested that magnets improve circulation, or that the electric current they generate interferes with pain signals. Proponents believe the magnets must be precisely placed to have the maximum effect, so magnetic therapy may be performed under the care of a doctor or health professional. Many people use magnets to self-treat pain, however; the benefit is unclear.

Magnets come in various shapes and sizes, from small strips that can be attached to the body to shoe insoles, mattress pads and car seats. The strength of a magnet is measured in gauss units – refrigerator magnets are about 60 gauss, while magnets sold for therapy are from 300 gauss to 4,000 gauss. Those that can be attached to the body range from 350 gauss to 500 gauss, while a magnetic mattress pad may be 4,000 gauss. People using magnets for pain relief may wear them for as little as five minutes or as long as several hours each day. No one is sure how strong a magnet must be to offer any benefit.

Prices range from $25 for small magnets to about $100 for magnetic insoles, up to $800 for a magnetic mattress pad. Experts say most low-level magnets are not beneficial and are a waste of money. You may want to buy any magnets from a vendor who offers a refund if it doesn't work for you.

SCIENTIFIC EVIDENCE

Magnets are just beginning to be studied for pain relief, and results are mixed. One often-cited study examined the effects of magnetic insoles on 19 people with peripheral neuropathy of the feet (pain caused by poor circulation) and found that participants reported pain relief. [Am Jour Pain Mgt 1999;9:9]

A double-blind, placebo-controlled study involving magnets for chronic pelvic pain also showed that participants wearing magnets for 24 hours a day for several weeks had some pain relief, [Am Jour Obstet Gynecol 2002 Dec;187(6):1581] but a study on low back pain found no effect on pain [JAMA 2000 Mar 8;283(10):1322].

A randomized, controlled trial using real and sham magnetic pads to treat fibromyalgia found that participants who had the real magnetic pads showed an improvement in pain intensity level, but other measures – tender point count and intensity, and functional status – were no different than the group that received sham magnets. [Jour Altern Complement Med 2001 Feb;7(1):53]

SIDE EFFECTS AND INTERACTIONS

- Magnets generally have few side effects.

- Some people note a tingling in the area of the body nearest the magnet.

SAFETY CONCERNS

- Magnets have not been tested on pregnant women, so their safety is not known.

- Do not use magnets if you have a pacemaker or implanted defibrillator, or near anyone who has these devices.

- Do not sleep on a magnetic mattress pad for more than eight hours.

- Turn off electronics that may be sensitive to magnetic fields, such as the switches on electric blankets.

Malic Acid

See Magnesium, page 176

Massage

Common uses:
Relieving pain, stress, stiffness

As a healing therapy, massage is ancient. Hippocrates, the father of medicine and author of the Hippocratic oath all doctors take, used massage as a therapy as early as 430 B.C. There are many different massage techniques, originating from regions all over the world.

Massage involves manipulation of the soft tissue of the body, usually using touch. For people with fibromyalgia, massage can have both physical and emotional benefits – it can help stretch tense muscles, improve flexibility, and help lessen pain, stress and depression, and it feels good.

In other cultures, massage is one of the basic medical treatments. It is part of Indian ayurvedic medicine and is widely used in Europe and Asia. In the U.S., massage is one of the most commonly used CAM therapies. Rheumatologists often recommend massage for fibromyalgia and arthritis, and many rehabilitation programs and pain clinics include a massage therapist as part of the treatment team.

There are more than 100 kinds of massage, each using a different technique. Some types are more physical, using pressing and stroking to work on muscles, while others pay more attention to the Asian philosophy of balancing the flow of energy in the body.

You can also use massage appliances or aids, which come in a wide variety of styles for a wide range of prices. There are even massage chairs that provide gentle stimulation to muscle and joints. Ask your doctor or physical therapist to recommend a massage aid appropriate for your particular condition and use only as directed.

Here are some of the common forms of massage:

- Deep tissue massage: This technique involves applying firm pressure on deep muscle or tissue layers to relieve chronic muscle tension. The therapist's strokes may go against the grain and he or she may use fingers, thumbs and elbows. This technique can help tight muscles relax, but it can also cause soreness and is not for everyone.

- Myofascial release: This type of massage targets tension in the fascia, the connective tissue that sheaths muscles. Therapists apply gentle but steady pressure to stretch the fascia. It is often used for fibromyalgia.

- Reflexology: In reflexology, the therapist manipulates the feet, hands or ears to improve function throughout the body. The idea is based on the belief that energy flows through 10 channels or zones that run throughout the body, ending in the hands and feet. Each zone links parts of the body to specific areas on the hands and feet. Whatever the theory, reflexology is extremely gentle – the therapist applies pressure with the tips of fingers and thumb – and may be a choice for people who find other types of massage too painful.

- Shiatsu: Shiatsu is a specialized form of massage that focuses on balancing the body's life energy, or chi. According to this philosophy, chi flows along certain pathways or meridians in the body, and illness results when chi is blocked. Shiatsu (which means "finger massage") is related to acupuncture and acupressure; the therapist presses and holds certain points on the meridians to restore the flow of chi.

- Skinrolling massage: This technique has shown good results for some people with fibromyalgia, although it can be very painful at first. The therapist gathers a roll of your skin and moves across the underlying fascia to break any adhesions binding tissue layers and nerves. Some people with skin-fold tenderness who have withstood the pain of the first few sessions claim they get long-lasting pain relief.

- Spray and stretch: Another technique that some say is helpful for fibromyalgia, spray and stretch involves applying a coolant (such as flouri-methane) to a painful area. Then the therapist gently stretches the muscles in that area. Physical therapists and medical doctors often perform spray and stretch massage.

- Swedish massage: This is what most people think of as massage – a full-body treatment that includes stroking, kneading or shaking muscles to relieve tightness. It can be soothing or vigorous, and may also increase circulation to muscles and joints and encourage relaxation.

- Trigger point therapy: In trigger point therapy or neuromuscular massage, the therapist applies deep finger pressure on specific points to release knots of tension or pain that can trigger pain elsewhere in the body. It can be helpful for fibromyalgia, but it can be painful if the pressure is too strong. Make sure your therapist is aware of your body's reactions, and stop him or her if the pressure is too strong.

SCIENTIFIC EVIDENCE

Clinical studies on the benefits of massage vary, with some showing notable results and others showing less improvement. Studies do show massage can decrease levels of stress hormones in the body, ease muscle tension and spasms, and help the body release endorphins, the body's natural painkillers.

One placebo-controlled study compared the effects of massage on fibromyalgia using three groups: one received Swedish massage, one received TENS (transcutaneous electrical nerve stimulation) and one received sham TENS treatment. After five weeks, the massage group had fewer symptoms, including insomnia, pain, fatigue and depression. The TENS group showed similar changes, but not until after the final day of the study. [Jour Clinical Rheum February 1996;2(1): 18]

Massage is considered safe for most people and many people should find it therapeutic. However, you should speak to your doctor before trying any massage therapy to make sure the particular massage therapy is appropriate for your condition and that the massage therapist you intend to use is qualified. You may have to try different massage techniques until you find one that works best for you.

Generally, massage sessions are performed with you lying on a padded table or mat on the floor in a warm and quiet room. Before beginning, the therapist should ask you about any health conditions or sensitivities and go over your goals for the therapy. You do not have to disrobe completely for a massage session. Some people do prefer to disrobe completely to help the therapist reach the areas he or she is working on, and also prevents stains from oils or lotions. This choice is up to you.

You will have a large sheet to cover yourself, and the therapist will uncover only the part of the body being worked on.

Most massage sessions last from 30 minutes to an hour. The massage should not hurt – some people even become so relaxed they fall asleep during the massage. Massage can be expensive and may not be covered by your insurance policy. In some cases, a doctor's prescription may be necessary for some coverage.

Safety Concerns

- Massage generally is considered safe when performed by an experienced therapist. Talk to your medical doctor first to find out if there is any reason you should not try massage – some massage techniques can worsen high blood pressure, osteoporosis or circulation problems.

- Do not have a massage on inflamed joints, during a flare, or if you are coming down with an illness. Do not massage areas where your skin is broken, sore or painful.

- If you are pregnant, tell the massage therapist before the session.

- Massage can cause strong emotions, such as sadness or even tears, to surface as your body becomes totally relaxed. If these emotions persist, you may want to seek counseling.

Finding a Practitioner

Massage therapists are required to be licensed in some states, but not all. You can ask your medical doctor for a referral, or ask friends and family. Physical therapists and chiropractors often work with massage therapists and can make referrals. Professional organizations also provide names of therapists in your area.

National Certification Board
for Therapeutic Massage and Bodywork
(800) 296-0664
www.ncbtmc.com

American Massage Therapy Association
(847) 864-0123
www.amtamassage.org

Meditation

Common uses:
Relieving pain, illness, stress, anxiety

Meditation, a state of relaxed mental awareness, has its beginnings in early religions. It has been a part of almost every religion in the world, used by spiritual seekers to attain a state of enlightenment. In the U.S., prayer is the best-known form of meditation. But you can get the same health benefits from practicing meditation without any religious component – it is the process itself that relaxes you.

There are many different kinds of meditation that use a number of awareness practices to focus the mind and body. The process involves sitting in a quiet place and concentrating your attention on an object, thought or sensation (it could be a sound, a word, your breathing or an image). Another kind of meditation involves cultivating "mindfulness" or awareness of the present moment. This approach, which begins by cultivating a single point of focus and expands to include awareness of thoughts, feelings or changing sensations in the body, is taught in many stress-reduction programs. In all forms of meditation, you allow any thoughts or feelings to arise and pass without becoming attached to them or focused on them. When your attention wanders, you gently bring it back to focus on the object, thought or sensation.

Some people meditate alone, others in a group. Some people meditate for pain relief or relaxation. Other people pursue meditation for its spiritual component. The length of each person's meditation also varies: Some people meditate for as long as a hour a day, although for a beginner even 10 minutes a day can show results. You gain the most benefits when you meditate every day. Some people find it helpful to have an instructor guide them through the process, but you can easily learn meditation techniques from books or audiotapes.

SCIENTIFIC EVIDENCE

Many studies show that regular meditation can benefit overall health, and that the benefits can be lasting. Researchers believe meditation may decrease activity in the sympathetic nervous system (which controls the body's reaction to stress), leading to decreased heart and respiratory rates, and lower blood pressure. Some studies have suggested that meditation lowers cortisol levels in the blood and encourages relaxed brain waves.

It is especially effective for fibromyalgia, particularly when combined with other mind-body therapies. A 1993 uncontrolled study of people with fibromyalgia found that all showed improvement in symptoms after a 10-week meditation-based relaxation program. [Gen Hospital Psychiatry 15, 284-289, 1993] Another uncontrolled study that combined an eight-week mindfulness meditation program with qi gong and pain-management techniques showed that people with fibromyalgia experienced improvement in pain threshold, depression, coping and function, and a follow-up study indicated these benefits lasted at least four months. [Altern Ther Health Med 1998 Mar;4(2):67]

SAFETY CONCERNS

- Meditation is a safe and inexpensive therapy. Some experts believe that excessive meditation can uncover suppressed emotions, so it helps to choose an experienced instructor.

- Some people find it difficult to sit still long enough to learn the technique. They may find that meditating while walking can help.

- If you feel uncomfortable with a particular type of meditation or instructor, stop and leave. If one type of meditation doesn't work for you, there are many to choose from.

FINDING AN INSTRUCTOR

Instructors are not certified or licensed in the U.S. It is taught at hospitals, spiritual centers, by mental-health professionals and at meditation centers. Make sure to ask about training and qualifications when choosing an instructor. Mental-health professionals are, of course, licensed to do therapy, and some incorporate meditation into their practices.

Melatonin

Common uses:
Treating insomnia, jet lag

Melatonin is a hormone secreted by the pineal gland, a pea-sized gland located deep within the brain. It regulates your biological clock, controlling the sleep/wake cycle and secretion of reproductive and digestive hormones. Melatonin release is stimulated by darkness and inhibited by light, telling the body when to sleep and when to wake up, and our bodies make less of the hormone as we age.

Most melatonin supplements are synthetic versions of the natural hormone. It is often used to relieve insomnia and jet lag and is not addictive. Since fibromyalgia is related to sleep disturbances, some people with the condition take melatonin to sleep better.

In Canada, France, Great Britain and other countries, melatonin is sold only by prescription.

Scientific Evidence

Some studies have shown that melatonin is effective for treating jet lag – it appears to help the body reset its internal clock across time zones – and for helping people who do shift work to restore normal sleeping patterns. Other studies have shown that melatonin is an effective sleep aid, especially in the elderly and people who have low levels of the hormone. It seems to shorten the time needed to fall asleep and to reduce the number of times people wake up during the night.

The evidence for fibromyalgia is more mixed. Various studies have indicated that people with fibromyalgia have too little melatonin [Clin Endocrinol 1998 Aug;49(2):179], too much [Jour Rheumatol 1999 Dec;26(12):2675] or the same amount as people without fibromyalgia [Jour Rheumatol 1998 Mar;25(3):551]. A 1998 study showed that women with fibromyalgia slept better after a nightly dose of the hormone, and an open study in 2000 found that that tender points decreased and participants slept better. [Clin Rheumatol 2000;19(1):9]

Melatonin has also been promoted as an anti-aging supplement, but there is no evidence that melatonin has this beneficial effect in humans.

SIDE EFFECTS AND INTERACTIONS

- People who take 3 mg or less of melatonin seem to experience few side effects.

- Melatonin may cause drowsiness about 30 minutes after taking the hormone.

- Other side effects include headache, stomach upset, lethargy and disorientation.

- Some people report feeling groggy upon waking, vivid or unpleasant dreams, and a worsening of insomnia.

- High doses may disrupt the body's internal clock and alter production of other hormones. They may also alter women's menstrual cycles and affect fertility.

- Melatonin interacts with a number of drugs and supplements. Taking the hormone along with sedatives, antihistamines, muscle relaxants and narcotic pain relievers can cause excessive drowsiness. These include benzodiazepines such as diazepam (*Valium*), temazepam (*Restoril*) and lorazepam (*Ativan*); barbiturates; narcotics; antidepressants such as fluoxetine (*Prozac*); antihistamines; and alcohol, as well as herbs such as valerian, chamomile and kava, among others.

- Melatonin can increase blood pressure and heart rate in people taking antihypertensive medications, including beta-blockers such as propranolol (*Indural*) and atenolol (*Tenormin*), as well as nifedipine GITS (*Procardia XL*).

SAFETY CONCERNS

- While melatonin appears to be relatively safe for short-term use, there is no evidence of its safety or effectiveness in long-term use. Melatonin is a hormone and can have wide-ranging effects. Talk with your medical doctor before taking melatonin, especially if you also take prescription drugs.

- Do not take melatonin with prescription corticosteroids or if you use birth control pills.

- Avoid melatonin if you have kidney disease, epilepsy, diabetes, depression, an autoimmune disease, serious allergies, heart disease, leukemia or multiple sclerosis.

- Do not drive or perform hazardous tasks after taking melatonin.

- Pregnant and breast-feeding women should avoid melatonin. Do not give melatonin to children or teenagers, as they naturally produce high amounts of the hormone in the body.

DOSAGE

A recommended dose is 1 mg before bedtime. Doses as low as 0.1 mg have produced a sedative effect in people with low levels of melatonin, so try a lower dose first. Buy supplements that contain synthetic melatonin; supplements made from animal glands pose the risk of contamination.

Milk Thistle (Silybum marianum)

Common uses:

Treating liver disorders such as cirrhosis and hepatitis; protecting the liver from toxins

Milk thistle is related to the sunflower and grows throughout the U.S. and other parts of the world. The seeds have been used for medicinal purposes dating back to the time of the Greeks and Romans. The active ingredient in milk thistle, silymarin, consists of three flavonoid compounds known as silymarin (silybin, silidianin and silichristine) that have anti-oxidant properties and also protect the liver by increasing glutathione, an amino acid-like substance that helps the liver neutralize drugs.

Some experts suggest buying supplements that contain milk thistle bound to phosphatdycholine, a component of the fatty compound lecithin, because the combination may be more easily absorbed than milk thistle alone. Milk thistle appears to be most effective when taken between meals.

SCIENTIFIC EVIDENCE

Many studies, mainly in Europe, suggest that milk thistle may improve cirrhosis and hepatitis. [Drugs 2001;61(14):2035] A major study in the U.S. is underway examining the use of milk thistle to treat hepatitis C. Milk thistle is also a powerful anti-oxidant, more potent than vitamins C or E.

People with fibromyalgia may take milk thistle to protect the liver from the effects of other drugs or supplements. In addition to processing nutrients, the liver helps the body neutralize many drugs, including acetaminophen (*Tylenol*), butyrophenones, phenothiazines and phenytoin (*Dilantin*), as well as alcohol. By increasing the amount of glutathione by as much as 35 percent, it is thought that milk thistle may protect the liver from damage.

SIDE EFFECTS AND INTERACTIONS

• Milk thistle generally has few side effects. Some people may experience loose stools, which can be counteracted by increasing the amount of fiber in the diet.

- Milk thistle may lower blood sugar levels, so people taking oral drugs or insulin for diabetes, or suing supplements that may also affect blood sugar levels (such as bitter melon) should have their blood sugar levels closely monitored by their medical doctor.

- Because milk thistle may interfere with the way the liver processes some drugs, anyone who takes prescription medication should talk with their medical doctor before taking milk thistle and should be monitored when using the herb.

- Anyone with an allergy to plants in the aster or thistle families should not take milk thistle.

- People with liver disease should not take milk thistle without first talking to their medical doctor.

SAFETY CONCERNS

- Milk thistle generally is considered safe.

- The herb is sometimes suggested to nursing mothers as a way to improve the flow of breast milk, but safety in pregnant and breast-feeding women has not been established.

DOSAGE

The common dosage for milk thistle is based on its silymarin content, with a suggested dose of 70 mg to 210 mg of silymarin three times a day, or up to 250 mg of standardized extract containing 70 to 80 percent silymarin.

MSM (methylsulfonylmethane)

Common uses:
Treating arthritis, back pain, muscle pain

MSM is an organic sulfur compound that's found in tiny amounts in blood and most foods. Sulfur makes up part of three amino acids in the body, and works with the B vitamins to help nerve cells communicate. It is an important nutrient for joints, and research has suggested that people with arthritis have lower amounts of sulfur in their joints then healthy people. Studies have shown that people who bathe in waters high in sulfur (See hydrotherapy, p. 162) get some relief from arthritis symptoms.

MSM has been proposed as a treatment for arthritis; it may have pain-relieving properties and anti-inflammatory effects, and help maintain and repair cartilage. So far, however, these claims are based on anecdotal evidence, not scientific study. Researchers don't know how MSM works once it gets to the joints.

MSM is made from DMSO (dimethyl sulfoxide), an industrial solvent that is approved as a treatment for interstitial cystitis. DMSO has a bad smell and is potentially toxic, but it is believed that MSM avoids those problems.

People with fibromyalgia may take MSM to relieve muscle pain. Because there is so little information about this supplement, many of its effects – and the long-term safety of its use – are unknown.

SCIENTIFIC EVIDENCE

There is very little scientific evidence about MSM; most of the suggestions for its use are based on how sulfur works in the body. One animal study indicated that MSM lessens joint damage [Patol Fiziol Eksp Ter 1991 Mar-Apr;(2):37] and most studies show few side effects or toxic dangers. [Altern Med Rev 2002 Feb;7(1):22]

SIDE EFFECTS AND INTERACTIONS

- Because MSM has not been studied much in humans, the long-term effects of use are unknown. Some people experience stomach upset, diarrhea and headache.

- MSM may have a blood-thinning effect and should not be used with anticoagulants such as warfarin (*Coumadin*), aspirin, or supplements with similar effects such as ginger or ginkgo biloba.

- So far, no allergies to MSM have been reported. Some experts warn people with allergies to sulfa drugs and sulfites to avoid MSM as a precaution, but others say MSM is safe even for people with allergies.

SAFETY CONCERNS

- MSM appears safe, but the lack of scientific studies means that some of its effects may be unknown.

DOSAGE

Most people who take MSM do so at a dose of 500 mg twice or three times daily. Take the supplement with meals to avoid stomach upset.

NADH (Nicotinamide adenine dinucleotide)

Common uses:
Treating depression, fatigue, Parkinson's disease

NADH is a coenzyme that the body makes from vitamin B3 (niacin). As their name suggests, coenzymes help enzymes work properly; enzymes are proteins that act as catalysts to change other substances in the body, such as changing food into energy.

NADH is used by the brain to make certain neurotransmitters and stimulates the production of ATP, which helps release energy in cells. Normally the body makes all the NADH it needs. Since some researchers believe an ATP deficiency contributes to fibromyalgia, NADH has been suggested as a supplement that may lessen fatigue and boost energy.

SCIENTIFIC EVIDENCE

Most of the uses suggested for NADH are based on how it works chemically. For example, because it helps produce L-dopa, which the body converts into dopamine, it has been proposed as a treatment for Parkinson's disease. Likewise, it has been suggested that NADH may help relieve symptoms of chronic fatigue syndrome by boosting energy.

Few studies have been done looking specifically at NADH's effects on these conditions, however, and most do not have scientifically reliable results. One randomized, double-blind, placebo-controlled crossover study indicated that NADH may be effective in treating chronic fatigue syndrome. [Ann Allergy Asthma Immunol 1999 Feb;82(2):185]

SIDE EFFECTS AND INTERACTIONS

- Not much is known about possible side effects or interactions with other drugs or herbs.

- High doses of NADH may cause nervousness, anxiety and insomnia.

SAFETY CONCERNS

- NADH appears safe, but the consequences of taking it long-term have not been established. Some experts recommend taking NADH for no more than four months, stopping for a month, and then resuming. Another option might be to take NADH two or three times a week instead of daily.

- Because of the lack of research, pregnant and breast-feeding women should not take NADH without first talking to their medical doctor.

DOSAGE

A common dose of NADH is 5 mg a day. Some experts recommend starting out with a lower dose and gradually increasing the amount taken over several weeks. Take NADH on an empty stomach.

Noni Fruit (Morinda citrifolia)

Common uses:
Relieving pain, inflammation, digestive problems

The noni plant (also called Indian mulberry) is native to Polynesia, where it has been used to treat a variety of illnesses.

Although different parts of the plant are used in Polynesia, in the U.S. the tree's four-inch, potato-shaped fruit is the part used for medicinal purposes. It has a bitter taste that is masked in commercial juices or supplements.

Noni is promoted for a wide variety of conditions and illnesses, including fibromyalgia – so much so that it seems to be claimed as a panacea for whatever ails you. But noni fruit has barely been studied at all in humans, so there is no evidence that it works. The best guess, based upon the fruit's properties, is that it may serve as a digestive aid.

SCIENTIFIC EVIDENCE

Almost no studies have been done on noni fruit in humans. Like most fruits, noni contains vitamin C, B vitamins, beta-carotene, potassium, amino acids, sodium, magnesium, iron, calcium and phosphorus. In addition, some chemicals found in noni fruit have been studied in the laboratory, where test-tube and animal tests indicate they may have pain-relieving, anti-inflammatory and anti-cancer properties, as well as some mild sedative action. [Acta Pharmacol Sin. 2002 Dec;23(12):1127] But whether any of these effects occur in humans is questionable.

Noni's reputation as a digestive aid comes from the fact that it contains anthraquinones, plant chemicals that relieve constipation.

SIDE EFFECTS AND INTERACTIONS

- Because of the lack of human tests, not much is known about noni's side effects. Nausea and stomach upset are possible.

- Theoretically, noni can increase levels of potassium in the body. People with kidney disease and those taking potassium-sparing diuretics should not drink noni juice.

- Some herbalists suggest that you do not take noni juice with coffee, tobacco or alcohol.

SAFETY CONCERNS

- Not much is known about the safety of noni juice. People with diabetes may want to avoid noni juice, as its effects on blood sugar levels are not known.

- Noni juice has not been evaluated in pregnant and breast-feeding women, so they may want to avoid the fruit.

- The smell and taste of noni juice can be unpleasant. Dried capsules avoid the problem, but it is not known whether the drying process changes noni's effectiveness.

DOSAGE

A suggested dose is 4 ounces of the juice taken one half hour before breakfast and on an empty stomach.

O-p

Passionflower (Passiflora incarnata)

Common uses:

Treating insomnia, anxiety

Passionflower is native to Latin and South America and was used by the Aztecs for pain relief and as a mild sedative. One of the active ingredients in passionflower is harmine, a compound that produces mild euphoria and was used by the Germans in WWII as a truth serum. Harmine can reduce the breakdown of the neurotransmitter serotonin in the body, which may have the effect of promoting sleep and pain relief.

SCIENTIFIC EVIDENCE

Most studies involving passionflower have been animal studies, which seem to indicate that passionflower has mild sedative effects. One recent study that compared passionflower to oxazepam (*Serax*) for treatment of anxiety found that both were equally effective. [J Clin Pharm Ther. 2001 Oct;26(5):363] However, most human studies for anxiety have used passionflower in combination with other herbs, such as valerian, so the effect of passionflower alone is not known. Passionflower is often combined with valerian in commercial supplements.

SIDE EFFECTS AND INTERACTIONS

• Because passionflower has not been studied much in humans, its side effects are unknown.

- In rare cases, there have been reports of skin rash, asthma-like symptoms and irritated sinuses. However, some herbalists believe these side effects were caused by contamination of the supplements.

- In theory, passionflower can increase the side effects caused by sedatives or antidepressants, notably drowsiness and low blood pressure.

- Do not combine valerian with benzodiazepines such as diazepam (*Valium*), temazepam (*Restoril*) and lorazepam (*Ativan*); barbiturates; narcotics; antidepressants, including MAO inhibitors such as tranylcypromine (*Parnate*), tricyclic antidepressants such as amitriptyline (*Elavil*) and selective serotonin reuptake inhibitors such as fluoxetine (*Prozac*); antihistamines; or alcohol without talking to your medical doctor. Passionflower may also increase the side effects of some herbs, such as valerian, kava and chamomile.

- Passionflower may increase the risk of bleeding when used with anticoagulants such as heparin or warfarin (*Coumadin*), NSAIDs such as aspirin, ibuprofen (*Advil, Motrin, Nuprin*) or naproxen sodium (*Aleve*). Similar effects may occur with herbs that have anticoagulant properties, such as ginkgo biloba and ginger.

- Caffeine combined with passionflower may raise blood pressure.

SAFETY CONCERNS

- Because passionflower has not been studied much in humans, its safety is not known.

• Pregnant and breast-feeding women should avoid passionflower, as its safety has not been studied.

DOSAGE

A suggested dose is 300 mg to 450 mg of powdered
extract in pill form 30 minutes before bedtime. Choose a
product standardized to 2.6 percent flavonoids. If you take
passionflower in a tincture, be aware that the preparation
may contain alcohol.

Phosphatidylserine

Common uses:

Treating Alzheimer's disease, "fibro fog"

Phosphatidylserine is a phospholipid, a kind of fat found
throughout the body but particularly concentrated in the
brain, where it keeps cell membranes fluid. It is believed to
help keep the memory-related pathways in the brain working properly. Because levels of phosphatidylserine decline
with age, it has been proposed as a treatment for Alzheimer's
disease and age-related dementia. Some studies indicate it is
effective, but although it is also touted as a treatment for the
mental fatigue that sometimes accompanies fibromyalgia,
no one knows whether it works in healthy people.

Phosphatidylserine is found in some foods (mainly rice and
leafy vegetables), but only in small amounts. Supplements
offer a more concentrated dose. Until a few years ago, phos-

phatidylserine supplements were made from cow's brains, but concerns about mad cow disease have caused manufacturers to shift to soy lecithin. Most scientific studies on the effectiveness of phosphatidylserine were done on earlier supplements, and it is not know whether soy lecithin is effective.

SCIENTIFIC EVIDENCE

Most studies of phosphatidylserine have focused on its potential as a treatment for Alzheimer's disease. It shows promise in slowing the mental deterioration associated with the disease, but it seems most effective in the early stages and benefits lessen as the disease progresses. [Dementia 1994 Mar-Apr;5(2):88] It also appears effective in treating age-related memory loss and mental functioning. [Aging (Milano) 1993 Apr;5(2):123] and preliminary research indicates it may help alleviate depression in the elderly. No studies have evaluated phosphatidylserine's effect on fibromyalgia.

SIDE EFFECTS AND INTERACTIONS

- Phosphatidylserine has few side effects. The most common are stomach upset and insomnia. To avoid these problems, take the supplement 30 minutes before meals and avoid any late afternoon doses.

- Some evidence suggests that phosphatidylserine may increase the risk of bleeding when taken with anticoagulant drugs such as heparin (*Calciparine*).

- People who take anticoagulants should not take phosphatidylserine without talking to their medical doctor.

SAFETY ISSUES

• Phosphatidylserine generally is considered safe.

DOSAGE

A suggested dose is 100 mg twice a day.

Polarity Therapy

Common uses:

Improving posture, reducing muscle tension

Polarity therapy is based on the belief that vital life energy, ruled by two opposite poles of electromagnetism, saturates the human body. Disease or illness results when this energy becomes blocked or misdirected. Restoring the balanced flow of energy leads to health and well-being. The therapy was developed by Randolph Stone (1890-1981), an osteopath, chiropractor and student of Eastern medicine.

To bring the body energy into balance, polarity therapy uses many methods and techniques from both western and eastern medicine, such as acupuncture, chakra balancing, postures similar to yoga, psychological counseling, bodywork or therapeutic touch, and nutritional counseling.

Polarity practitioners use touch to guide the flow of energy (the right hand is thought to carry a positive charge, the left hand a negative one) by placing the hands on soft tissues and energy points. The practitioner may use varying degrees of pressure: either a "neutral" touch (light), a "positive" touch (stimulating) or a "negative touch" (deep), though usually the majority of bodywork involves only a light touch.

The diet suggested in polarity therapy is usually vegetarian, though specific recommendations depend on the illness being treated. Some foods may be added or eliminated from the diet based on ayurvedic principles of a person's personality type (ether, fire, air, water or earth — see Ayurvedic medicine, p. 84).

At your first visit to a polarity practitioner, he or she will take a detailed medical history and ask about your diet, exercise program, home and professional life, and general mental and emotional well-being. The practitioner will also perform a hands-on examination of your energy flow. Each session will include some bodywork, but other therapies such as nutritional or psychological counseling are only given as needed.

A similar therapy is reiki, a Japanese technique involving a practitioner placing his or her hands on various parts of the body in order to relieve pain, stress and tension. Reiki is a Japanese word meaning "universal life energy," and reiki practitioners believe that they are helping to transmit healing, spiritual energy into the recipient of the therapy. Reiki sometimes is lumped in with types of massage (see p. 182), but practitioners claim that their therapy is not massage, as they do not knead muscles and other tissues.

SCIENTIFIC EVIDENCE

There is no scientific evidence to suggest that polarity or other therapeutic touch techniques work, and little clinical study of these therapies. Most research concerning therapeutic touch has focused on whether "energy fields" exist around the body. One double blind study in 1990 found that skin wounds treated with non-contact therapeutic touch healed quicker than those not treated with therapeutic touch. The study investigated whether non-contact therapeutic touch had any effect on the healing of skin wounds. [Jour Subtle Energies 1990;1(1):1-20]

However, a 1998 study asked therapeutic touch practitioners to identify which of their hands was closest to an investigator's hands, to test whether they could correctly identify an energy field emanating from the investigator. Practitioners correctly identified the position of the investigators hand 44 percent of the time, no better than the result expected by random chance. [JAMA 1998 Apr 1;279(13):1005]

SAFETY ISSUES

- Polarity therapy and similar therapeutic touch therapies generally are considered safe.

- People with fibromyalgia may want to ask the practitioner to avoid any firm-pressure touch.

FINDING A PRACTITIONER

Polarity practitioners are not licensed; however, the American Polarity Therapy Association certifies practitioners who have completed 155 hours of coursework to be

associate practitioners and 460 additional hours to be registered polarity practitioners. The association provides a list
of practitioners in your areas; contact the APTA at (303)
545-2080 or on the Web at www.polaritytherapy.org.

Q-s

SAM or SAMe (S-adenosylmethionine)

Common uses:

Easing depression; treating fibromyalgia, osteoarthritis, migraine headaches

SAM or S-adenosylmethionine is a compound produced by the body from methionine, a sulfur-containing amino acid, and adenosine triphosphate (ATP), an energy-producing compound. SAM is involved in a number of biochemical reactions in the body. It helps in forming neurotransmitters, including dopamine and serotonin, and aids in maintaining levels of glutathione, a major anti-oxidant that protects cells from damage.

Used for some time in Europe to treat arthritis and depression, it is marketed in the U.S. under several names, the most common being SAMe.

SCIENTIFIC EVIDENCE

SAM has been the subject of a number of scientific studies. An analysis of clinical controlled studies showed it was as effective as tricyclic antidepressants in relieving mild to moderate depression, and that it worked faster (often within a week) and had fewer side effects. [Acta Neurol Scand Suppl 1994;154:7]

SAM has also shown promise in treating the symptoms of fibromyalgia. Several studies have shown a reduction in the number of tender points and amount of pain, as well as improvement in mood, in people with fibromyalgia who took SAM. [Am Jour Med 1987 Nov 20;83(5A):107] However, a 1997 study using intravenously administered SAM did not show significant benefits. [Scand Jour Rheumatol 1997;26(3):206]

Studies involving thousands of people with osteoarthritis have shown that SAM can increase joint mobility and reduce swelling and pain about as well as NSAIDs, and without the risk of side effects such as stomach bleeding. Preliminary animal studies suggest it may help repair cartilage.

SAM can be expensive. Weigh this factor when you are considering using SAM as a supplement for treating a chronic disease like fibromyalgia.

SIDE EFFECTS AND INTERACTIONS

- SAM generally has few side effects. Large doses may occasionally cause stomach upset, nausea or insomnia.

- People with bipolar disorder should not take SAM, as its antidepressant properties may lead to mania.

- If you take antidepressant or anti-anxiety drugs, do not take SAM without talking to your medical doctor first – the combination may increase side effects.

SAFETY CONCERNS

- SAM generally is considered safe.

DOSAGE

A recommended dose is 200 mg to 400 mg twice a day. Experts suggest buying enteric-coated pills, and taking

SAM on an empty stomach between meals. To avoid insomnia, don't take SAM late in the day. Folic acid and vitamin B12 are needed for SAM to work in the body, so experts suggest getting enough of these nutrients in your diet or taking a supplement that includes them.

Note: Do not treat severe depression with SAM. Depression is a serious illness and should be treated by a medical doctor.

St. John's Wort (Hypericum perforatum)

Common uses:
Treating anxiety, insomnia, fibromyalgia

St. John's wort is a shrubby perennial plant with small yellow flowers that is grown all over the world and is known as the "natural *Prozac*." Supplements are produced from the dried flowers, which contain the chemicals hypericin and hyperforin.

Scientists aren't sure exactly how St. John's wort works, but it may boost levels of the neurotransmitter serotonin, which affects mood, pain and well-being. It is the most widely prescribed antidepressant in Germany and one of the best-selling supplements in the U.S. A recent study has called into question the efficacy of St. John's wort for treating moderate depression, and a study to see whether it is effective for mild depression is planned.

SCIENTIFIC EVIDENCE

Evidence about St. John's wort's efficacy is mixed: While a number of studies over the last 20 years have shown that St. John's wort is effective in treating mild to moderate depression, a recent study by the National Institutes of Health showed it was no better than placebo for treating major depression of moderate severity. However, the study also indicated that sertraline (*Zoloft*), a serotonin reuptake inhibitor (SSRI) was no better than placebo in relieving primary symptoms of depression. [JAMA, 2002; 287:1807] The study's authors note that in 35 percent of studies of approved and active antidepressants, the antidepressants do not show greater effect than placebo.

In previous studies St. John's wort appeared to be as effective in treating depression as tricyclic antidepressant drugs and has fewer side effects. [BMJ 1996 Aug 3;313(7052):253]

St. John's wort is often suggested for people with fibromyalgia and chronic pain. Although scientific studies do not show a lot of evidence for these uses, people with fibromyalgia often have low levels of serotonin, which may be boosted by taking St. John's wort. In addition, depression often accompanies fibromyalgia.

SIDE EFFECTS AND INTERACTIONS

- St. John's wort generally has few side effects; most studies show St. John's wort has no more side effects than placebos. The most common include constipation, stomach upset, sedation, restlessness, dry mouth and increased skin sensitivity to sunlight.

- People taking St. John's wort were once advised to avoid the same foods avoided by those taking MAO inhibitors, such as cheese and red wine. However, recent studies indicate that those foods pose no risk to people taking St. John's wort.

- St. John's wort may affect the way certain drugs are broken down by the liver, leading to increased or decreased levels of the drugs in the blood. Specifically, St. John's wort may lower levels of protease inhibitors, tricyclic antidepressants such as amitriptyline (*Elavil*), cholesterol-lowering drugs, digoxin, and theophylline; and may increase levels of SSRIs and MAO inhibitors. If you take medications or other supplements, talk to your medical doctor before taking St. John's wort.

- If you take antidepressant or anti-anxiety drugs, do not take St. John's wort without talking to your medical doctor first – the combination can cause increased side effects.

- St. John's wort may increase skin sensitivity to sunlight when taken with other drugs with the same effect, such as tetracycline and tretinoin (*Retin-A*).

- If you take birth control pills, use St. John's wort with caution – there have been reports of bleeding and unwanted pregnancies.

SAFETY CONCERNS

- St. John's wort generally is considered safe. It can take four to six weeks to be effective. If your symptoms do not improve, or if you experience severe depression, see your medical doctor right away.

• Do not treat moderate or severe depression with St. John's wort. Depression is a serious illness and should be treated by a medical doctor.

• Pregnant and breast-feeding women should avoid St. John's wort, because the herb has not been studied in this group.

DOSAGE

A common dose is 300 mg of St. John's wort standardized to 0.3 percent hypericin, taken three times a day. Take the herb at mealtime to reduce stomach upset.

T-v

Tai Chi and Qi Gong

Common uses:
Easing inflexibility, anxiety, pain, stiffness

Tai chi is a series of movements and positions developed in China that address both the body and the mind. It began in China in the 1200s as a form of martial arts and is a popular for of exercise in China today.

Tai chi is designed to balance and enhance *qi* (pronounced chee), the vital life energy that flows through every living thing. Qi is the guiding principle of Chinese medicine (see Chinese medicine, p. 112), which holds that disease occurs when qi is blocked or out of balance. Both tai chi and qi gong are believed to stimulate qi, promote self-healing and improve the functioning of the body.

There are many different styles of tai chi and qi gong, all based on meditation and gentle movements drawn from nature or animals. In tai chi, you perform a sequence of slow movements combined with deep breathing and mental focus. The series of positions flow together into one long movement. These movements keep the body stable while its weight shifts. All movements are performed slowly and without force, and have poetic names such as "part the wild horse's mane." They can be lovely to watch.

Qi gong is similar, but the movements are made up of short sequences that are held for a few seconds and repeated. Some movements involve only the arms. The goal is to become aware of and direct the flow of qi throughout the body.

Many rheumatologists recommend tai chi or qi gong as an excellent form of exercise for people with fibromyalgia, because their gentle movements build muscle strength without stressing joints. Some find qi gong easier to perform, especially if muscle aches in the legs and hips are a problem. People of all ages and at all fitness levels can perform tai chi and qi gong.

To learn either discipline, take a class. Don't try to learn by watching a videotape. It's important for an instructor who has been trained to show you how to do the movements properly. Some instructors also have experience teaching people with fibromyalgia or arthritis. Look for a beginners' or senior citizens class, and tell the instructor you have fibromyalgia. Once you learn the basics, you can practice on your own. A short form of tai chi takes about 10 minutes and includes 24 movements; the long form can take 40 minutes and includes more than 100 movements.

Tai chi classes usually begin with warm-up exercises, then breathing techniques or meditation to focus the mind. The instructor demonstrates movements and the class follows. Sequences are repeated, with students focusing on movements, bathing and inner balance. Qi gong classes are similar.

Tai chi and qi gong do not provide an aerobic workout.

SCIENTIFIC EVIDENCE

No specific studies examining tai chi's effect on fibromyalgia have been completed. Many Chinese studies speak of the benefits of tai chi and qi gong, but few Western studies have been done. One uncontrolled study of fibromyalgia used qi gong in combination with mindfulness meditation and found that participants reported improvements in depression, pain threshold, coping skills and function following the study and even lasting four months. [Altern Ther Health Med 1998 Mar;4(2):67]

SAFETY CONCERNS

- Tai chi and qi gong are considered quite safe. Just about anyone can do them. Because even gentle exercises can be harmful if not done correctly, make sure you find a qualified instructor and tell him or her about any physical limitations.

- Find your own pace, and do only as much as feels comfortable. Most instructors believe that the internal focus on qi is more important than the actual physical exercise.

FINDING AN INSTRUCTOR

There is no licensing or training requirement to be an instructor in tai chi or qi gong, so you may have to do a bit of research. Ask your medical doctor or physical therapist for a referral, check with community centers or health clubs, or contact a traditional Chinese medicine center. The Qi Journal Web site also has a list of instructors at www.qi-journal.com.

Valerian (Valeriana officinalis)

Common uses:

Treating insomnia, anxiety; promoting restful sleep

Native to North America and Europe, valerian is a perennial plant with pink flowers whose root has been used as a sedative for centuries. The root contains a number of compounds, including valepotriates and valeric acid, which are thought to bind to or enhance brain receptors for a neurotransmitter called gamma-aminobutyric acid (GABA) to promote sleep. That action is similar to how diazepam (*Valium*) and other benzodiazepines work, but valerian is not addictive and does not cause grogginess the next morning. Rather than inducing sleep, valerian appears to relax the brain and body so you can go to sleep.

In Germany, Great Britain and elsewhere in Europe, valerian is approved by health officials as a sleep aid. Because sleep disturbance is one of the hallmarks of fibromyalgia, people with the condition may take valerian to promote restful sleep – there is some evidence it can prevent people from waking up frequently during the night.

Valerian has an unpleasant odor and taste. Gel-caps or capsules may be the best way to take the supplement, although it is available in tea form.

SCIENTIFIC EVIDENCE

Several studies suggest that valerian can reduce the amount of time it takes to fall asleep and can improve sleep quality. In one study, participants were given an over-the-counter supplement of valerian mixed with other ingredients, valerian alone, or a placebo. Those taking valerian alone fell asleep more quickly and woke up during the night less often than those taking either placebo or the combination. In addition, valerian was most effective for those who had the greatest sleep problems. [Pharmacol Biochem Behav 1982 Jul;17(1):65]

Some early evidence also suggests that valerian may be effective as an anti-anxiety agent, but most studies have involved valerian combined with other herbs. [Fundamental Clinical Pharmacology 1997; 11: 127]

SIDE EFFECTS AND INTERACTIONS

- Valerian generally has few side effects when used at recommended doses.

- Rarely, headache, decreased ability to concentrate, dizziness, lower than normal body temperature and stomach upset have occurred.

- In theory, valerian can increase the side effects caused by sedatives (notably drowsiness). Do not combine valerian with benzodiazepines such as diazepam (*Valium*), temazepam (*Restoril*) and lorazepam (*Ativan*); barbiturates; narcotics; antidepressants such as fluoxetine (*Prozac*); antihistamines; or alcohol without talking to your medical doctor. Valerian may also increase the side effects of some herbs, such as St. John's wort.

- Although valerian does not appear to cause drowsiness per se, one German study indicated it did impair performance for several hours after participants took the herb. Avoid driving or doing anything hazardous after taking valerian.

SAFETY CONCERNS

- Valerian generally is considered safe. It has only been studied for four to six weeks' use, so the effects of long-term use are not known.

- Pregnant and breast-feeding women should avoid valerian, as its safety has not been studied.

DOSAGE

A recommended dose is from 150 mg to 300 mg of powdered extract in pill form 30 minutes before bedtime. Choose a product standardized to 0.8 percent valeric acid. You can safely increase the dose to 600 mg to 900 mg if the above has no effect.

Visualization

See Guided Imagery, page 158

Vitamins

Common uses:
General health and wellness

Vitamins are essential for good health. In fact, the body needs 13 vitamins to function properly – A, C, D, E, K, and the B vitamins (thiamin, riboflavin, niacin, pantothenic acid and biotin, vitamin B6, vitamin B12 and folate). Although the best way to get the vitamins your body needs is by eating a healthy diet, most people fall short of that ideal. In addition, some people with fibromyalgia believe that taking more than the Recommended Daily Allowance (RDA) of some vitamins can help alleviate their symptoms.

Recent research has helped promote the anti-oxidant properties of some vitamins, and in some cases larger doses are touted as doing everything from warding off cancer to slowing aging. But not all vitamins are safe in large amounts – and scientific studies have yet to show that additional amounts of vitamins truly benefit healthy people.

With that said, below are some of the more popular vitamin supplements taken for fibromyalgia.

Vitamin C (water-soluble, anti-oxidant)

Common uses:
Boosting immune system; healing wounds; easing colds and other infections; easing asthma; preventing cataracts, certain cancers

Most animals make their own vitamin C, but humans have to get it in their diet. It's the most popular vitamin supplement in the U.S., extensively researched for its anti-oxidant properties. One of the things vitamin C does is help produce collagen, an essential protein found in con-

nective tissues, cartilage and tendons. A high dose of vitamin C has been associated with a decreased risk of
osteoarthritis. People with fibromyalgia often take extra C
in the hope that it can lessen muscle damage and pain. The
"Meyer's Cocktail," an intravenous supplement of vitamins
and minerals that contains magnesium, calcium, B vitamins, and vitamin C, has also been suggested as a treatment
for fibromyalgia, but it has not been clinically evaluated.

SCIENTIFIC EVIDENCE

A study published in 2000 suggested that vitamin C may
have beneficial effects for people with fibromyalgia, though
the study was small and not rigorously designed. Twelve
women with fibromyalgia who took a 500 mg-blend of
ascorbigen and broccoli powder for one month reported
less sensitivity to pain and better quality of life. [Altern
Med Rev 2000 Oct;5(5):455]

SIDE EFFECTS AND INTERACTIONS

- Vitamin C has few side effects. The body excretes what
  it does not use, so even high doses aren't toxic. However,
  doses above 2,000 mg can cause mouth ulcers, diarrhea,
  gas and bloating.

- High doses of vitamin C may increase the body's absorption of aluminum from certain antacids such as *Maalox*
  or *Mylanta*. Take vitamin C at least two hours before taking an antacid.

- Vitamin C increases iron absorption and decreases the
  absorption of copper.

- At high doses, vitamin C may decrease the body's ability to excrete acetaminophen (*Tylenol*), and theoretically could allow dangerous levels to build up in the blood.

- Taking vitamin C with tetracycline may increase levels of the antibiotic in the body.

SAFETY CONCERNS

- Vitamin C is considered safe, even at high doses. The body can only use 1,000 mg per dose of vitamin C, so anything above that in a single dose is not beneficial.

- People on dialysis, or those with kidney stones, kidney disease or gout should avoid high doses of vitamin C, which may increase the formation of kidney stones.

- People with hemochromatosis, a disease that results in too much iron in the body, should not take vitamin C supplements.

DOSAGE

A suggested dose is 500 mg of vitamin C daily.

B Vitamins (water-soluble)

Common uses:
Relieving fatigue, depression; promoting healthy skin, eyes, hair, other organs

The B vitamins include eight vitamins – thiamin (B1), riboflavin (B2), niacin (B3), pyridoxine (B6), folic acid (B9), cyanocobalamin (B12), pantothenic acid (B5) and biotin – and are involved in many processes in the body, including energy production, digestion and functioning of the nervous system. They work together, so are often taken as a B-complex supplement.

Some studies have suggested that people with fibromyalgia may have lower levels of the B vitamins, [Scand J Rheumatol. 1997;26(4):30 and J Adv Med 1992;5:105] and many of the symptoms of vitamin B deficiencies are similar to the symptoms of fibromyalgia (confusion, muscle fatigue, depression, and numbness or tingling in hands and feet). A deficiency in vitamin B6, for example, can cause problems with sleep, and low levels of B6 have been associated with stress and anxiety. Many people with fibromyalgia take extra doses of B6 and B12 to help combat fatigue. (See also NADH, p. 198.)

SCIENTIFIC EVIDENCE

Most of the studies done so far attempt to correlate a deficiency in B vitamins with the symptoms of fibromyalgia; no studies show that taking B vitamin supplements can reduce symptoms. One study showed that injections of B12, an often-used treatment by medical doctors for fatigue, had no effects on chronic fatigue syndrome. [Arch Intern Med. 1989 Nov;149(11):2501]

SIDE EFFECTS AND INTERACTIONS

- Thiamin (B1): No significant side effects. Sulfites (food preservatives) and black tea may lessen the effectiveness of thiamin. Some drugs, including diuretics such as furosemide (*Lasix*), can cause thiamin deficiency. Magnesium is needed to convert thiamin to its active form (and thiamin is often included in magnesium/malic acid supplements).

• Riboflavin (B2): No significant side effects. Riboflavin interacts with some chemotherapy drugs, birth control pills, antibiotics and psychiatric drugs, so check with your medical doctor before use. Riboflavin is needed to convert B6 into its active form.

• Niacin (B3): Niacin can be toxic in large doses. Side effects include flushing of the skin, stomach upset, nausea and liver damage. Do not take niacin without first talking to your medical doctor. Niacin may increase the effects of cholesterol-lowering drugs such as atorvastatin (*Lipitor*), gemfibrozil (*Lopid*), lovastatin (*Mevacor*), pravastatin (*Pravachol*) and simvastatin (*Zocor*), causing muscle pain and kidney damage. Do not take niacin if you also take these drugs. Niacin can affect blood sugar levels, so people with diabetes should not take niacin without talking to their medical doctor. Also avoid niacin if you have low blood pressure, glaucoma, gout, liver disease or ulcers, and do not take time-release niacin – it seems to affect the liver more.

• Pantothenic acid (B5): No significant side effects. High doses may affect the body's absorption of biotin and cause diarrhea. A suggested dose is between 100 mg and 500 mg per day, taken with meals.

- Pyridoxine (B6): High or moderate doses of vitamin B6 can cause nerve damage when taken for long periods of time – most experts recommend a dose of no more than 50 mg per day. Vitamin B6 may reduce the effectiveness of anti-convulsant drugs such as phenytoin (*Dilantin*) and pheno-barbital. People taking levodopa (*L-dopa*) should not take B6 unless it is combined with carbidopa, as in *Sinemet*.

- Folic Acid (B9): Large doses may causes seizures in people with epilepsy, and are dangerous for those with hormone related cancers. High doses can cause gas, nausea and loss of appetite. A high intake of folic acid can mask a B12 deficiency and vice versa, so most people take these vitamins together.

- Cyanocobalamin (B12): No significant side effects. A high intake of folic acid can mask a B12 deficiency and vice versa, so most people take these vitamins together. Vitamin B12 interacts with a number of drugs, including antibiotics, methyldopa (*Aldomet*), azidothymidine (*AZT*), birth control pills, cimetidine (*Tagamet*), metformin (*Glucophage*), famotidine (*Pepcid*), soprazole (*Prevacid*), omeprazole (*Prilosec*), and rantidine (*Zantac*). A high dose of 1000 mcg per day is sometimes recommended for fibromyalgia, either taken as an injection given by your medical doctor or possibly as a sublingual tablet.

- Biotin: No significant side effects. Very high doses may affect insulin requirements in people with diabetes.

Vitamin E (fat-soluble, anti-oxidant)

Common uses:
Preventing heart disease, cancer; anti-aging aid

Vitamin E is a powerful anti-oxidant that has been proposed as a treatment for everything from cancer to heart disease to osteoarthritis. A fat-soluble vitamin, vitamin E actually includes eight related compounds – tocopherols and tocotrienols, in four different forms, alpha, beta, delta and gamma. Natural and synthetic vitamin E are available; some experts recommend natural vitamin E (d-alpha-tocopherol) or natural mixed tocopherols.

Because most of the sources of vitamin E in foods are high in fat, many experts recommend a vitamin E supplement as part of a healthy diet; people with fibromyalgia make take extra E to combat pain and boost immunity.

SCIENTIFIC EVIDENCE
Vitamin E's role in treating heart disease has been well studied. The Cambridge Heart Anti-oxidant Study found that people with existing heart disease who took vitamin E lowered their risk of heart attack by 77 percent compared with those who took a placebo. [Lancet 1996 Mar 23;347(9004):781]

Evidence for pain relief in fibromyalgia and other rheumatic diseases is mixed. An older study published in 1942 suggested that vitamin E did lessen pain in people with "fibrositis." [J Bone Joint Surg 1942;24:411] But a study in

2001 comparing vitamin E to placebo found no effect on pain in people with osteoarthritis. [Annals of the Rheumatic Diseases October 2001;60:946]

SIDE EFFECTS AND INTERACTIONS

- Vitamin E generally is considered safe even at high doses. Possible side effects include nausea, gas, diarrhea, heart palpitations and increased bleeding.

- Vitamin E interacts with a number of drugs and supplements. Because of its blood-thinning properties, it can increase the effect of anticoagulant drugs such as warfarin, heparin, aspirin and herbs such as ginger and gingko biloba. People who take these drugs and supplements should talk with their medical doctor before taking high doses of vitamin E.

- You should stop taking vitamin E before any surgery.

- Vitamin E may affect the effectiveness of tricyclic antidepressants and antipsychotic drugs such as chlorpromazine.

- Cholesterol-lowering drugs such as atorvastatin (*Lipitor*), gemfibrozil (*Lopid*), lovastatin (*Mevacor*), pravastatin (*Pravachol*) and simvastatin (*Zocor*) may reduce the anti-oxidant properties of vitamin E.

DOSAGE

A common dose is 400 IU twice daily.

W-z

White Willow Bark (Salix alba)

Common uses:

Easing pain, inflammation

The active ingredient in white willow bark, which comes form the white willow tree, is salicin, a chemical relative of acetylsalicylic acid, the ingredient in aspirin. In fact, salicin was the starting point for the development of aspirin (aspirin was created from a different herb called meadowsweet).

White willow bark is often called "herbal aspirin." In the body, salicin is converted to salicylic acid, which lowers levels of prostaglandins (inflammatory compounds). White willow bark acts similarly to aspirin, although not as fast, and causes fewer side effects such as stomach bleeding.

Choose pills rather than teas made from white willow bark because the dosage is more reliable (the bark contains only 1 percent or less of salicin, meaning you would have to drink several quarts of tea to get a useful dose). Choose extracts standardized to 40 mg salicin.

SCIENTIFIC EVIDENCE

White willow bark has been used for thousands of years to treat headaches and fevers. Today it is used to relieve headaches, muscle aches, menstrual cramps and inflammation from arthritis. Most scientific studies have examined white willow bark in combination with other herbs, so there is not much evidence of the effect of white willow bark by itself.

SIDE EFFECTS AND INTERACTIONS

- White willow bark seldom causes side effects at suggested doses. Higher doses may lead to stomach upset or tinnitus (ringing in the ears). If you experience any of these side effects, stop taking the herb immediately.

- Anyone who should avoid aspirin – people who are allergic, those with ulcers, teens or children with fevers – should also avoid white willow bark.

- Do not take white willow bark if you have tinnitus.

- Do not take white willow bark with aspirin or NSAIDs, because the combination can increase the risk of stomach bleeding.

SAFETY CONCERNS

- Never give white willow bark to children under 16 who have symptoms of cold, flu or chickenpox. Although the herb is metabolized differently than aspirin, there is a chance of developing Reye's syndrome, which can be fatal.

- Pregnant and breast-feeding women should avoid white willow bark.

DOSAGE

A standard daily dose is 60 mg to 120 mg, divided into three doses.

Yoga

Common uses:

Improving flexibility, relaxation

Yoga is an ancient practice involving breath control, meditation and exercise that combines mental, physical and spiritual training. Yoga is offered at many health clubs and even physical rehabilitation centers all over the U.S., and millions of people at all levels of fitness and of all ages practice yoga everyday.

Yoga places as much emphasis on mental health as it does on physical fitness (the word "yoga" means union in Sanskrit). Research indicates that yoga can help lower blood pressure, increase energy and may even help relieve mild depression. It can also improve flexibility, increase muscle strength and balance and encourage relaxation.

There are several kinds of yoga, including *bhakti*, which focuses on spirituality, and *hatha*, which is most popular in the U.S. And there are several schools of hatha yoga, ranging from gentle stretches to vigorous workouts. All involve carefully held positions, called *asanas*, and slow, regulated breathing techniques, called *pranayama*. Positions (or poses) include standing, sitting and prone postures, all performed with attention to breathing and your body's sensations.

Yoga can be an excellent form of exercise for people with fibromyalgia, because of its emphasis on stretching and meditation, and on letting students go at their own pace.

To learn yoga, take a class – don't try to learn by watching a videotape. It's important for an instructor who has been trained and certified to show you how to do the postures properly. Some instructors also have experience teaching people with fibromyalgia. Look for a beginners' or senior citizens' class, with a slow pace and an instructor who modifies the positions based on each student's ability, and tell the instructor you have fibromyalgia.

A yoga session usually begins with breathing exercises, which help the body relax and the mind free itself from distractions. Yoga students learn how to concentrate on taking long, deep breaths through the nose and then exhaling. Some gentle overall stretches may be next, and then the instructor will begin the postures. They usually include standing postures, balance postures, and backbends or twists.

Standing postures help improve balance and increase lower body strength; poses done sitting or lying down will increase muscle strength and flexibility. The instructor will demonstrate each pose first and then check to see that each student performs it properly. Not all students will be able to mimic the instructor's pose, and that's perfectly acceptable – the instructor will help you modify the poses or use a rolled towel or pillows, so you can move as far into the pose as is comfortable for you.

A yoga session usually ends with a brief meditation or deep relaxation exercise. People who meditate regularly say it helps them sleep better, increases concentration and memory, and improves general well-being. Although there are more claims than case studies for yoga and meditation, it is a safe, accepted way to relax and focus the mind.

Yoga classes generally last from an hour to 90 minutes. Though a weekly class helps you make sure you are performing the poses correctly, it is important to practice yoga daily to get the full benefits. A basic routine can take from 15 minutes to an hour. You can do yoga at any time of day, though it's best to avoid any exercise right before bedtime. Most forms of yoga do not provide an aerobic workout.

SCIENTIFIC EVIDENCE

No specific studies examining yoga's effect on fibromyalgia have been done. A few studies have suggested that yoga can help relieve anxiety [Jour Personality Clin Studies 1989;5(1):51], alleviate depression [Indian Jour Clin Psychology 1993;20:82] and increase general well-being. One study found that pranayama (breathing techniques) resulted in a greater feeling of alertness compared to relaxation and visualization techniques and that a daily 30-minute yoga routine had an invigorating effect on mood and physical energy.

SAFETY CONCERNS

- Yoga generally is considered quite safe. Just about anyone can do it. Because even gentle exercises can be harmful if not done correctly, make sure you find a qualified instructor and tell him or her about any physical limitations.

- Ask your medical doctor if there are any poses you should avoid. If your doctor isn't familiar with yoga, take a book that has pictures of the poses with you to your appointment.

FINDING AN INSTRUCTOR

There is no licensing requirement to be a yoga instructor, although individual yoga schools do certify instructors who go through teaching programs. You can ask your medical doctor or physical therapist for a referral, or talk to people who have taken a class. Many health clubs and senior centers offer classes. You can ask the instructor if he or she has any experience working with people with fibromyalgia. You can also visit a class before signing up.

The American Yoga Association does not offer referrals, but it provides good information about the history and types of yoga. Contact the organization at (921) 927-4977 or on the Web at www.americanyogaassociation.org.

Zinc

Common uses:
Boosting immune system, relieving pain, treating illness

Zinc is an essential mineral found in every cell of the body, used in almost every enzyme reaction and needed to make many body hormones function properly. It is particularly important for the immune system, and to help wound healing and keep skin healthy. Many Americans do not get enough zinc in their diet.

Autoimmune diseases, including fibromyalgia, lupus and rheumatoid arthritis, may be linked to zinc deficiency, and zinc has been demonstrated to affect pain in animal studies. People with fibromyalgia often have lower levels of zinc in the body, and it has been suggested that taking zinc supplements may help to relieve pain. Zinc lozenges have also gained popularity as a treatment for colds and flu.

SCIENTIFIC EVIDENCE

Zinc has been studied most extensively as a treatment for colds, and the evidence is mixed: Some studies show that zinc lozenges can shorten the duration of a cold, while others show no effect. [J Nutr 2000 May;130(5S Suppl):1512S] A study by Dr. I. Jon Russell specifically examined zinc and fibromyalgia, and found that although zinc levels were lower in people with the condition, the levels rose only slightly after supplementation and there was no effect on pain. The study concluded that that zinc deficiency may contribute to fibromyalgia pain, but that zinc supplements cannot yet be recommended. Some evidence also suggests that people with inflammatory bowel disease have lower levels of zinc, and that supplementation may help reduce symptoms. [Aliment Pharmacol Ther 1993 Jun;7(3):281]

SIDE EFFECTS AND INTERACTIONS

- Taking zinc in amounts greater than 200 mg per day can cause nausea, vomiting and diarrhea. Taking 100 mg per day long-term can lower levels of HDL ("good") cholesterol, suppress immune-system function and cause anemia. Talk to your medical doctor before using zinc for more than a week.

- Zinc may decrease effectiveness of antibiotics including tetracycline, doxycycline, ciprofloxacin and minocycline. Take zinc at least two hours after these antibiotics.

- High doses of iron or calcium can decrease the amount of zinc absorbed in the body.

SAFETY ISSUES

- Some research indicates that too much zinc may be associated with Alzheimer's disease, but further study is needed.

DOSAGE

A suggested dose is 30 mg per day. Your total intake of zinc – including food and supplements – should not exceed 150 mg per day.

Conclusion

Now you have a great deal of information about CAM therapies and how they may play a role in your self-management of fibromyalgia. Some therapies may be helpful, others may be useless and some may be harmful to your health. The most important tool you have in your effort to control fibromyalgia symptoms is knowledge. Credible information can be hard to find. We hope this book offers you some useful, solid information about the treatments you are curious about and will help you make decisions about what to do next in your search for treatments.

This book was developed in response to the growing number of people being diagnosed with fibromyalgia and the proliferation of information about CAM therapies on the Internet, in magazines and more. There is a great deal of conflicting and unsubstantiated information about CAM treatments for pain, muscle aches and other symptoms of fibromyalgia. This situation only creates confusion and anxiety for people with chronic illness – people who obviously have many other sources of stress to deal with. It is our hope that this book and other resources of the Arthritis Foundation will clear up some of the confusion, lessen the anxiety and offer you credible information about the therapies available to you.

This book is not a substitute for your doctor's directions or advice, nor is it our intent to guide you or influence you in your decisions about CAM. Only you and your doctor can decide whether or not you should use CAM treatments, and what treatments you should investigate. This book is meant to be another, solid source of information.

RESOURCES

For more information about the Arthritis Foundation, call our toll-free number, (800) 283-7800, or visit our Web site, www.arthritis.org. Both resources contain a wide variety of information for people with fibromyalgia, chronic pain and arthritis-related diseases. Find the Arthritis Foundation chapter office closest to you through these avenues, and explore the many resources chapter staffs and volunteers have to offer in your community.

The mission of the Arthritis Foundation is to improve lives through leadership in the prevention, control and cure of arthritis and related diseases.

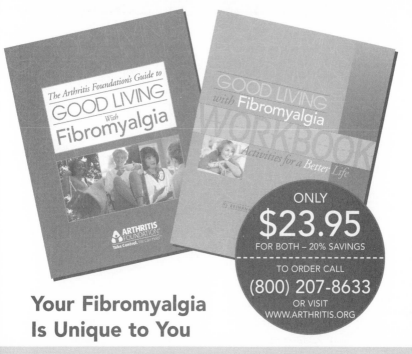

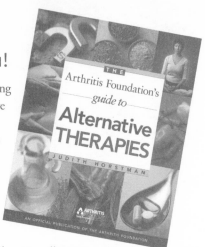
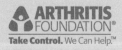